God Spoke I Listened

by
Randy B. Brown

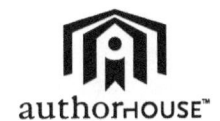
authorHOUSE™

1663 LIBERTY DRIVE, SUITE 200
BLOOMINGTON, INDIANA 47403
(800) 839-8640
WWW.AUTHORHOUSE.COM

First published by AuthorHouse 09/21/05

ISBN: 1-4208-3869-5 (sc)
ISBN: 1-4208-3868-7 (dj)

Library of Congress Control Number: 2005902172

Printed in the United States of America
Bloomington, Indiana

This book is printed on acid-free paper.

Stories and prayers by: Randy B. Brown
Poems by: Thelma Conway
Editors: Anne Chick, Ana Nehring, and Carol Piotrowski
Date: July 2005

ALL GLORY TO GOD!

Romans 8:28 "And we know that all thing work together...
according to His purpose."

These stories and poems are God's. He gave them to my mother
and me during our quiet times. Through the Holy Spirit, God gave
me every word on these pages as He put the poems and stories
together. They are revelations of His creation on earth.
Open your heart to accept what He has to tell you. Open your
eyes to His unique ways so He may have your attention and reveal
Himself to you in an intimate and personal way.

To HIM we give all the Praise, Honor, and Glory!
Thank you, my Jesus.

DEDICATION

To: A very special lady

Sister Jane Lowder: The day we were personally introduced you
asked if you could pray for me. While holding my hands you said,
"Your hands are beautiful. God says you will write poems and
little stories for Him." You did not know then, but this book was
already in progress. The title was "God's Little Stories". God
used that prophetic word to inspire me to finish this book. He
re-titled it, "God Spoke I Listened". Thank you, Sister Jane, for
your love and dedication to God and His Word. "WONDERFUL,
WONDERFUL JESUS!"

Also to: My Pastors

Pastor Chris and Pastor Miriam Phillips: God has seated me under
your spiritual leadership for the last ten and a half years. You have
depth of wisdom and pure unconditional love for your congregation
such as I have never seen in anyone. You have been a blessing to
my family and me in our spiritual walk and I am blessed to have
both of you as my Pastors. May the Lord continue to fill you with
wisdom, knowledge, strength and love as you continue to serve
Him. Thank you, Pastor Chris and Pastor Miriam!

Also To: My Husband of Thirty-Two years

Allen went home to be with the Lord in 2004. He loved me in spite
of all my faults. With his whole heart, he took care of our family.
Allen taught me what unselfish love is.

Also to:

My Three precious children: Rob, Crystal, and Angel. You continue to put joy in my life. It would not be complete without any of you. I am blessed to be your mother. Thank you for always being there for me. I love you so much!!!!

Also To:

Kristi (Daughter-in-Law), James and Stacey (Sons-in-Laws): You have loved and blessed my children and you have given me your unconditional love and support. I love you all! Thank you for your love and support.

To my ten precious grandchildren:

Chase, Chelsea, James, Matthew, Robbie, Ashley, Courtney, Eliyah, Charlie, and Miriam. You bring life into my home and you make me feel young again. I love you all so much!

Also to: My Mother and Father

Thelma, my mother, went home to be with the Lord in 1999. She inspired me with her faith and God given gifts. She wrote all the poems I have put in this book. Mom titled her Book "POEMS, MY GIFT FROM GOD."

Bob, my father, went home to be with the Lord in 1999. His character of freely giving to others inspired me. He was the most honest person I ever knew.

Also to:
My Best Friends

Anne Chick. You are not just my editor, but, most importantly, my mentor. Because of your wisdom and patience, I have discovered a personal, intimate relationship with Jesus I never knew existed. Thank you, Anne for your devotion to this book. Thank you for your love and support.

Ana Nehring. God used you not only to help edit this book, but He brought you into my life at a very difficult time. You supported me through the battles and helped me to laugh again. Thank you for helping with this book and all your love, support and laughter.

Mary Harris. You have such godly wisdom it is a blessing to everyone. Your kind, gentle and sweet spirit humbles me all the time. God also brought us together as friends during a difficult time in my life and I praise Him for your friendship and love. Thank you for your laughter, love, and support.

Also to a Few Very, Very, Special Friends:

Jackie Hornage, Jay Hill, Evelyn LaBonte, Quinn Slack, Karen Slack, Marilyn Nakamura, Terrance Gamble, Kathy Peterpaul, and Carol Piotrowski. You have all walked with me these last few years through many difficult trials and battles. You show what a loyal and loving friend truly is. Thank you all for the friendship, support, and love.

Index

Introduction

My relationship with God is priceless and very precious. I believe when we talk to God, He talks back to us in many different and unique ways. One way He talks to me is through my eyes. It does not matter what I look at; God will reveal Himself to me through his creation.

Sometimes it can be the simplest thing. I am worrying about something and thinking about it as I am driving. A car will drive by and I notice the tag reads 'W I L Y-100'. Immediately my spirit will hear God asking me, *"__Would I leave you__? No, I am with you __one hundred Percent__!"* I hear God's voice through the Holy Spirit, taking that acronym on the tag, giving me a message of encouragement. He shows me things that need to change in my attitude and character as well as reminding me of His word hidden deep inside my heart. As long as I am open to His voice, God will reveal Himself through what my eyes see. As you read these stories, you will see how God uses everyday things to get my attention. My grandchildren, my dogs, or favorite numbers I have, are only a few things He used in an unusual way to reveal His presence. He will speak through something I am eating, showing me things that need to change within my own heart.

Look around; see God's creation; hear all that He has to say to you. Be still and know that it is God *(Psalm 46:10)*. His Word says, "My sheep know my voice...follow me" *(John 10:27)*. God created all things *(Genesis 1:1, Colossians 1:16)*. I have learned to talk to Him as if He were sitting right next to me. His presence is so overwhelming, so peaceful I do not want to leave it. You too will want to stay and listen as He reveals Himself to you *(Jeremiah 33:3)*, in ways that are meaningful only to you. God has so much to talk to you about.

When God sent Jesus into the world to be our Savior, it was to reconcile us back to Him. People quit listening to God. They became disobedient and sinful. They did not recognize all that He had given them. The commandments given to Moses *(Exodus 20:3-17)* were ignored and the world had lost all respect for the Creator.

God loves us so much that He sent His **ONLY** Son to be the final sacrifice, to die by the hands of mankind for our sins *(John 7:28-29, John 3:16-17)*. God's love is like nothing we understand love to be. I could never give one of my children up for anyone, let alone someone that did not respect me. His love reaches far beyond our comprehension could ever imagine. If we stop and give God reverence, He will reveal Himself to us. Keep your focus on Jesus and let the Holy Spirit guide you *(John 14:26)*. Be blessed and filled with joy and peace from the blessings of God and ALL His creation.

When my mother went home to be with the Lord, she left her book of poems to me. As I read them, I knew God had a purpose for them. I discovered that purpose when God put this book together. They are His revelations of creation that He wants to use to encourage us. This book is for God's glory and His purpose. Be blessed and encouraged in your relationship with the Father, the Son and the Holy Ghost as you read these stories, prayers and poems.

The book cover is an actual vision the Lord gave me one day as I was praying about not being worthy for God to hear my prayers, and asking Him if I even had enough faith in Jesus? I just needed to know

God was listening to my prayers because things were not happening in the time limits I put on my requests. I felt it was taking so long to hear an answer or maybe God just was not listening to me. I was not in an intimate relationship with the Lord at this time, like I am now, so it was hard for me to receive His grace and love. I have had many visions but this one was life changing for me and I felt it was the one God wanted me to use for the cover of this book.

The VISION:

I was standing in front of a podium that had a huge book laying on top of it. The book looked like the unabridged dictionary it was so big! I assumed it was the book of life. A being of light illuminated behind the podium and behind the light were these beautiful gates made out of marble and pure gold. The gates were close. As I stood with my arms stretched toward the light, Jesus was standing to my left and a little bit behind me. I could feel the Holy Spirit's presence on my right, but I could not see Him. All of a sudden, the light began reading from the book. Each time the light said something to me, Jesus would stand in front of me and said, "I paid for that with my Blood". Than He would, step back until the next page was turned and the light spoke again. This went on page after page as the light went through the whole book. Jesus did and said the same thing each time. When the last page of the book was read, Jesus stood in front of me, and once again said, "I paid for that with my Blood". After that, the light closed the whole book, the gates opened up wide, and the being of light said to me, "Now you are worthy to enter the gates". I knew at that moment, we are not worthy, only Jesus is worthy! Because of our trust and faith in Christ, one day we will be changed in His image, than we will be worthy to enter the gates of heaven for all eternity.

Theirs nothing we can do, or anything we ever have done, that makes us worthy, except for the Blood of Christ that covers our sins. God hears our prayers. Just pray the way Jesus taught His disciples to pray. We pray to the Father, in the name of Jesus, believing in faith as we put our requests before God. God says we have not because we ask not. Jesus tells us to ask in faith, in His name, and it shall be given unto us. Yes, we are sinners, saved by grace, cleansed by the Blood of the spotless Lamb of God.

God loves us and He hears our prayers. We need to be patient and wait on His answers. We do not always hear when we want to. However, God does answer but in His time. So be patient, pray in the name of Jesus, have faith, and believe what you are praying. God is listening. He loves you with an unconditional love and it is His will that you live an abundant life. One filled with love, joy, and peace, forgiven by the Blood of Christ.

Sherika Hagans, a friend of mine, drew the picture. She listened as I describe the vision to her. Sherika has a wonderful gift of hearing something, the Holy Spirit gives her the image, and she can draw exactly what you are telling her. I am thankful for her God given talents and gifts. I pray that the cover and the meaning behind it will encourage you in the Lord, as it did me.

I pray God's love will fill your soul when you open your heart and see for yourselves the unique ways God speaks to you with revelations of who He is. The relationship you develop will be the most precious and priceless gift you will ever have. As you draw closer, God will give you those personal revelations of who He is and you will have a personal, intimate, relationship of love with your Father in Heaven.

I thank my Father in heaven, my Savior, and Holy Spirit, for all

He has done, is doing, and will continue to do in each one of us. I pray that as you allow God to use you to bless others you will feel the joy of the Lord. I know I do every time I get to share something that God has done in my life. *(ACTS 20:24 - But my life is worth nothing unless I use it for doing the work assigned me by the Lord Jesus.......Good News about God's.....love)*.

Some of the names in this book have been changed to protect people's privacy while some of the names are of actual people, used with their permission.

All scriptures are from different Bible translations I read, but you can read whichever one you have. God's Word is truth and will never pass away (Luke 21:33).

Randy B. Brown

Written By: Thelma Conway
21 September 1999

This is the last poem my mother ever wrote.
It was for my boss, Jay Hill. This Poem is
about his blessed earthly father who was
taken home to be with the Lord.

Dear Jay

Your Dad walked up the Golden Stairs,
Where Jesus was waiting for him there.

The Pearly Gates sprang open wide –
As the Lord brought your Dad inside.

The Trumpets were blowing a beautiful sound,
As the 'Angels' danced round and round.

There is no night in Heaven, we know
Just wonderful days watching flowers grow.

Walk "In the Garden" and talk to the Lord each day
Keeping your Dad close as you go on your way.

Hold on to "Precious Memories" and the good times you had.
Your Dad wouldn't want you to ever be sad.

We can look to Heaven and pray to the Lord above.
He will take care of you and fill you with His Love.

So "Turn your Eyes Upon Jesus" today,
He loves you so much and will show you the way.

We are children of the Heavenly Father, who loves us every day
So each time you lean on Jesus, His Son, do this and pray.

God please bless this son and let him know now –
You give him the strength to go on somehow.

Eternal Life

Jim's father was dying. The cancer was eating through his body, moving quicker than the doctors could handle. The devastation that Jim was feeling radiated from him. We sat across from one another that chilly morning in November, meeting over a cup of hot coffee. Jim's father, Jerry, had always been the stabilizing factor in Jim's life, the rock he leaned on. The imminent loss of his father was affecting everything about Jim. He no longer wanted to live. "My dad means everything to me," Jim said. "How can I live without him?" "Do I even want to live without him?" These were just some of the things tormenting Jim's mind as we talked.

As I thought about Jim's words, wondering how to respond, God spoke and I listened. **_Eternal life_** was the words I heard deep within my spirit that day. What does this mean, Lord? What I perceived as a loss forever is only a temporary loss. Life is full of temporary losses. As my children go off to the first day of school and as they leave home for college, I feel the loss. I continue on because I know it is only temporary. I know I will see them again. I continue with my work, missing them. When they return home, I find myself happy to see them, over joy for the time I get to spend with them before they leave again. It is only a temporary loss I am feeling.

Death seems so permanent at times like this we feel overwhelmed and it is hard to get our thoughts together. God gives us eternal life **_(John 10:28-29)._** Many times, we do not think about heaven and all of God's promises when we are walking through a trial of a dying loved one. We seem to think about one thing, how life is going to be for us without them. It is hard thinking about being without them every day. Of course, we are sad; it is a natural feeling God put inside of us. We do not understand all those feelings. I take nothing from those feelings Jim was having because it is not an easy trial to walk through, but what I heard the Holy Spirit say to me while trying to comfort him was how we need to lean on God's promises of eternal life.

Jim losing his father is heartbreaking and devastating. Dying is a loss hard for anyone to deal with. It is difficult to comfort friends during times like this because we do not know what to say to them. Jerry is saved and knows Jesus, and so does Jim. Even though Jerry was ready to go home to be with the Lord, it was hard for Jim to let go of his Dad. God understands our pain so He provided a way to comfort us through the Holy Spirit. Jesus left us the Holy Spirit so we would not be comfortless *(John 14:18, John 14:26-27)*. He gives us strength to walk through the trials and He gives us peace in our broken heart because of the encouraging words we hear from those who God has put there to support us through the battles.

Lately I had been witnessing to Jim about the joy of the Lord *(Nehemiah 8:10)*, telling him how Jesus would heal all his pain and wanted to comfort him now. This particular day though, Jim became very angry. He said he did not want to hear what God had to say about **JOY** or **PEACE** when his father was dying! My heart broke for him. I do not know what I would do without either one of my parents. The Holy Spirit was giving me words of encouragement to comfort Jim and I wanted to tell him the promises in God's word about eternal life *(John 10:27-30)*, but he walked away angry at the Lord. He did not understand why this had to happen to Jerry. We have salvation through the Blood of Christ and Jerry is born again *(John 3:3)*, walking with the Lord in his daily life. Jim walked away refusing to hear anything about God's peace. I did not understand how he was feeling but God knew his pain and felt his sorrow. All I could do was pray for God to help Jim through this time in his life.

The Bible says to fellowship with God and with one another *(I John 1:1-4)* so that our joy may be full. We encourage and remind each other what God's promises are; how He takes care of our pain during times like this, as well as anything we are experiencing. It is okay to be angry, but sin not *(Ephesians 4:26)*. It is okay to cry and weep. Jesus wept *(John 11:35)*. We cannot ignore what God wants to say to us during the tough times, however. There is healing in the Blood of Christ and we need to trust what God is saying through others to comfort us with His peace. God will send people to support and encourage us. They will speak the truth in God's Word and it will bring hope to our hopeless situation so our joy can be full in the Lord.

It seems all Jim has done lately is complain about everything. He is taking his pain out on everyone around him. He does not mean to, but he doesn't know what to do with all that pain inside him. He has temporarily unfocused his eyes off the Lord. God wants to heal all that hurt inside his heart. All Jim needs to do is stop, refocus his thoughts, and cry out to God. Jim is thankful that Jerry is saved and will be in heaven with the Lord, but the pain of losing his father makes it hard for him to concentrate. It hurts when we lose someone. What is important is that we know Christ as our Savior. We must try to have an open heart so we can receive what God is doing through others to comfort us. I felt when Jim walked away he had turned his back on God because of the pain he was feeling. Instead, I had longed for him to reach out to God and receive the peace the Lord wanted to give to him.

Although any loss is hard, we must not forget during times of pain and suffering how the Lord wants to comfort us. We need to reach for God, not turn away from Him. No one loves us as much as Jesus does. He said He would never leave us nor forsake us *(John 14:18, Hebrews 13:5)*. He is there right in the midst of all our pain. We must encourage each other to trust in the Lord, especially when we are hurting like Jim was. It is hard when we go through the death of loved ones but God is faithful and He will send someone to help us through the battle. We need to be open to His Spirit who dwells within us and receive His peace during times like this. We cannot tell God how we think He should comfort us. The scripture about Christians who will fall away from God in the last days *(Luke 8:13 and I Corinthians 15:58)* is very serious, especially during times of trials and suffering. We cannot turn our backs on God because we are angry at what is happening. God tests our faith *(Job 7:17-18)*. It is difficult in times of death and it is not an easy test, but we do have God's promises that give us comfort while we are walking through it.

Do not let the devil deceive you with your pain and cause you to turn your back on God because you are angry. Anger is only one way we can fall away from God. There are many other ways too, but this kind of pain is the most difficult to deal with because we have so many emotions running through us. It can cause us to be bitter, like having faith in God for some things but not for other things. Jesus says we either have faith one hundred percent or we are lukewarm and He will spew us out of His mouth *(Revelation 3:16)*. Jim could fall away from God because of the anger he is feeling at Him. This is the time for Jim to draw closer to God and receive comfort. We need to encourage each other and remember that we too, one day, because we are saved, will be with our loved ones, if they are saved.

I do not know Jim's heart, so we should also remember not to judge one another *(John 7:24, Matthew 7:1)*. God knows everything and He sees the deepest part of our heart *(1 John 3:20)*, so we should not judge each other because of what we see with our eyes.

God will take care of our broken heart. We have no idea what God has in mind for our future from one day to the next *(Matthew 6:34)*, but if we trust Him, He will take care of our hurts everyday. Yes, Jim hurts and I hurt for him. If my heart is aching for my friend how much more does our Heavenly Father's heart ache for Jim. Let us remember to encourage each other with God's promise of eternal life and as others share with us, we need to receive what God is speaking through them to comfort us. Remember we cannot pick and choose how we think God should be comforting us through the Holy Spirit. Just be open to the Lord and let Him do things His way. God's ways are everlasting. We cannot just be there for our friends and walk with them through battles. We need to encourage them in the Lord and let God put the joy back inside those empty and broken places in their heart. We too need open hearts to hear the Lord's voice inside us. God will use us as His vessels of love, peace, and joy in this world as He comforts others.

It is okay to hurt, to cry and to get angry, but remember, let the Lord bring the comfort, peace, and joy back into your broken heart. It is time we stop looking to the world to comfort our brokenness and reach to Heaven for God's comfort. Only He can heal us in a perfect way. Be open and receive what God is doing through others around you to encourage you. He may be using them to fill the emptiness you are feeling inside.

Christians love Jesus, they really do! However, some will choose worldly comfort over an eternal truth. They seek God for what He can do for them here on the earth but forget what He wants to do for them in eternity. They love and serve the world thinking because they go to church on Sunday they know Jesus. Many do not understand the power of the Holy Spirit and His purpose here on the earth. Some do not even know who the Holy Spirit is, while others are fearful to open up to the new things in God. Many just do not comprehend what they cannot see. They want all the facts and proof it is from God before they will listen, or even receive what God has for them.

Christians, we need to let our faith rise inside of us and speak with boldness what Jesus teaches us in the scriptures and what the meaning of eternal life is. We need to share that the Holy Spirit is real and what He does for us here. Jesus sits on the right hand of God but He left us the Holy Spirit so we would not be powerless and we would have all we need to live in this world *(Luke 24:49)*. It is the Holy Spirit's job to comfort us and He uses us as the vessels to serve the Lord here on earth. I know, in my life God does it all the time as long as I am open to His voice inside me and I do not just listen, but act according to His purpose.

We can learn something from all kinds of broken hearts. This story is just about one. Work at keeping your focus on God, the **CREATOR**. This is not the time to turn from God, but the time to run to Him for His plans of eternal life! Praise Jesus for the blood He shed on the Cross for our sins *(John 6:53-56)*! Start sharing God's truth about eternal life with others. Help people to realize worldly peace is only temporary, not something that is permanent. Only Jesus can heal our wounds in that perfect way. Encourage each other to reach for the Lord, not the world. Teach one another how to draw strength from the Lord, through the Holy Spirit's indwelling, by the living word of God that is hidden deep inside you. The Holy

Spirit will bring the scriptures to your remembrance and you can be a supporting friend and an encouraging vessel God has sent to your friends for that time in their life.

Jim has now walked through the loss of Jerry. God was with him because Jim reached for God's help before it was too late. He found peace and has accepted his loss because of the comfort only God could give him. Jim now has a testimony to share with others of God's peace and comfort when they may walk through the same fiery trial he has just come through. God will use Jim for many who will cross his path with that same type of hopelessness he was feeling, and he can share how God helped him to overcome it. I praise God for answered prayer. He does come quickly and heal the brokenhearted. All we have to do is pray and ask in the name of Jesus *(John 14:13-14)*. It is that easy.

At the time of that conversation with my friend Jim, my parents were still alive; however, a few years later I found out what that pain of hopelessness felt like. Both my parents died four months apart from each other. I remembered what the Holy Spirit taught me that day about eternal life. My parents were both saved and I know I will see them in heaven one day because I am saved too; but the pain was still hard to bear. I leaned on God for strength and He used Jim to encourage and comfort me this time. I have learned from my own experience to trust God with everything. He walks with us through all our trials and battles. We are not alone. We must not let the enemy deceive us with our anger or hopelessness we are feeling while walking through battles. It was pain and hurt Jim was feeling that day and not anger at all. I too felt the pain and hurt with my own battle. I learned from Jim's experience and I knew I had to trust my Father in Heaven to help me through it.

That day at the coffee shop was an experience of learning to lean on God's comfort as we walk through the trials in our lives. God will help you too if you just cry out to Him. Do not be afraid to tell God you are hurting and cannot understand all that pain and emotions you are feeling. He understands. Jesus is waiting to help you.

There are those who do not know Jesus. Christians, share the gospel with everyone, for one day we will be held accountable to God for what He has given us *(Romans 14:12)*. Jesus told us to go out and spread the gospel *(Mark 16:15)*. He did not tell us to keep it for ourselves and hide it from the world. Jesus tells us to "seek ye first the kingdom of God...all things shall be added unto you *(Matthew 6:33)*." I am glad the Holy Spirit revealed the truth to me about eternal life that day with Jim. It made my parents' death a lot easier to walk through. All the hurt and pain was there, but the comfort and peace of the Holy Spirit helped me get through as I opened up to the things God said through other people He put in my life to support me.

Let us pray:

Father, I thank you for Jesus, for your love and the power of the Holy Spirit that dwells within me. I thank you for the victory through the blood you shed on the Cross for all my sins, Lord. You are wonderful, mighty counselor, Prince of Peace and I praise you. Father, help me to seek you first when walking through any trials I am experiencing. Give me the strength to walk through the battles and trials in my life. Take away the pain of losing my loved ones and help me not to be angry at the world or turn my back on you during those times or any battle I am facing, in Jesus' name. Father, give me rest in my spirit. I know I am never alone, Lord; you are always with me. Father, I ask you to forgive me when I have failed to come to you first for comfort and peace. Forgive me, Lord, when I walk in my own strength and forget to lean on you. Holy Spirit, in Jesus' name, come, lead, guide, and direct my paths. Help me to receive the promises of comfort and peace when others try to encourage me, and help me to encourage them too. Father, be the thoughts in my mind and the words in my mouth when I share your promises with others about eternal life. Thank you, Father, for the things you do in and through me. Let me be an open vessel to share your love with others as you have commanded me to love one another as I love myself. I praise you and give you all the honor, Lord. In Jesus' name I pray.

Randy B. Brown

Written By: Thelma Conway
March 1955

My Children and I

My little children, and I have three
Are not so very much trouble to me?
One is six, one eight and one seven
Each one to me is a bundle from Heaven!
Each day, as I trudge off to work
While other duties at home I must shirk
Little arms around my neck embrace,
Begging, "Mamma" please don't go anyplace!

Two boys, a little girl, equally as sweet
Each one trying hard to compete
For the affection of Mom, their pride, their joy
Striving hard for a home for them to enjoy.
I love my children; they're my all, my heart
I pray each day nothing will tear us apart
They love me and though at times they're bad - -
I pray hard to God to get them a good Dad!
They now have a man, who'll soon a Daddy be
All the things they've missed, soon they'll see –
That someone in the world loves little ones near
To hold them to their heart and be sincere!
So thank You God! You've been so kind
At last you've given me peace of mind.
For now a family are we - -
Living in a home as it should be!

A Popcorn Heart

It was so cold outside that day in the middle of February 1997 and I did not want to go out for lunch, so I decided to eat at my desk. When I stay in my office during lunchtime, I have found that there is so much peace around me, alone with the Lord, in the middle of my busy workday. I can hear God's voice in the quietness of my office when I shut my door to the outside world. This particular day I was not very hungry, so I decided to eat some popcorn. I sat there munching away on popcorn and talking to God. The Holy Spirit filled the air as He began showing me some things about that popcorn sitting in front of me. I sat there listening to His voice inside me, not thinking about anything. I just wanted to be alone with the Lord and sit in His presence. He was right there in the midst of my little office. God's presence was all around me, while I was eating popcorn.

As I sat there looking at the popcorn in front of me, I begin to notice how some of the kernels were fully cooked, totally done, nice, and fluffy white. Some of them were not cooked at all and still in their kernel state. Others seemed to come close to being popped but they were only half-baked, and there were still others almost popped where you could see the whiteness peeking through but they were not puffed up enough yet to perfection so they were hard to chew. A specific piece God was showing me happened to be one that I thought was fully cooked with no flaws. I picked it up and bit down on it. To my surprise, there was a tiny piece of cornhusk hidden underneath its fluffy white shape that I could not see. As I bit into it, I just pulled it out, tossed it away, and went on eating more popcorn. God started telling me some things about that piece of popcorn and the hidden husk inside it. He said there are things in my own heart that were hidden and He wanted to change them. He saw things hidden inside me that I had covered up by my emotions and actions so others could not see how sad I really was. I knew they were there, and so did God, but no one else knew. The Lord continued speaking to me about how a Christian's heart can be just like this popcorn.

As I listened to Him speak into my spirit He revealed to me how at first we do not know Jesus until someone shares Him with us. When we come to Jesus and are born again *(John 3:3)*, we become a new creature in Christ, forgiven and cleansed, and we are now called a Christian. We start off full speed ahead on fire for Jesus because we want everyone to know Him like we do. We call that feeling our first love. We get so hot and puffed up we forget to stop along the way to get cooked with spiritual fillings. These are studying God's word, praying, going to church to hear the word of God spoken into our spirits by the pastor, and fellowshipping with other believers. Some of us are lying there just like a half-baked piece of popcorn. We are half-baked in His Word for living. Oh, we may begin to grow in the things of God, but we might not take the time to stop and get fluffy and perfected by the Holy Spirit's teachings in God's Word. There are others around us who look like they are working very hard on their faith. They will talk about studying the word, how they go to church all the time, and how they go to conferences, etc. However, there may be hidden deep down inside those hearts a stone God has not been able to crush yet, because they have not stopped to get fully cooked in the Word. They may not even know it is there because it is so deeply buried inside of them. Our human eyes will see these Christians as being popped to perfection in the Lord and in their faith, because we cannot see the hidden junk deep inside their heart and mind.

The Holy Spirit revealed to me *(Revelation 3:13)* what we are seeing with our eyes, as being popped to perfection in their spirits, still may not be perfectly popped and pure in God's eyes. If we do not recognize the convictions of the Holy Spirit, we cannot get fully popped or be able to confess all of our sins He is trying to show us. We may still have a stone stuck deep down inside the center of our heart. It may have some hidden hate, anger *(Ephesians 4:31)*, lies, bitterness, grudges, unforgiveness, lust, deceit or many other sinful things we are not even aware of. As a piece of popcorn could have a husk hidden beneath its beautiful fluffy white exterior, we too may look fluffy in the Lord with our smiles and good deeds. As we bite down into a piece of popcorn we feel the husk that is hidden and we pull it out, toss it away and go on eating more popcorn just like I did today. In this same way a Christian may also brush off things the Holy Spirit is convicting them of, toss them off and go on without really repenting and seeking forgiveness *(1 John 1:8-10)*, as if nothing is wrong with them. They may not confess these convictions before the Lord because they have not taken the time stop and listen to the Holy Spirit revealing what God wants to change inside their heart. They are walking in darkness thinking no one knows because they cannot see inside their heart or even know the way they really feel. God knows because nothing is hidden from Him *(Luke 16:15)*. You can hide things from the world but you cannot hide anything from God. He knows the very number of hairs on your head *(Matthew 10:30)*.

It is time to get rid of the tiny known and unknown sins hidden beneath the center of our heart. Be open to the convictions of the Holy Spirit, stop, and listen with an open ear as we go before our Father in Heaven seeking His forgiveness. Walk in the light, popped to perfection in Jesus and be careful to recognize convictions over condemnation. There is a difference and the enemy will try to steal your conviction and make you think you are doomed where God is concerned. Satan will condemn you and bring up the past to keep you from being free in Jesus. The Holy Spirit brings convictions so God can clean your heart from all sin. Jesus came not to condemn... but that we might be saved (John 3:17). We are free because of the Blood of Christ!

Remember, God sees through flesh and bone to the very center of our heart. Our heart needs to be popped to perfection with the Word of God in them. Get rid of those hidden sins. We can all have a fluffy, pure heart by receiving salvation through the Blood of Christ and letting the Holy Spirit guide us into all righteousness **(1 John 1:9)** and understanding the word of God.

The husk hidden inside the fluffy white piece of popcorn is in darkness just like the hidden sins within our heart is in darkness. God's Word says there is no darkness in Him *(1 John 1:5)*. Talk with God in prayer, confess your sins, and ask Him to reveal the unknown sins to you so you can confess them also. Remember, we can hide from the world, but we cannot hide from God. Take each day and spend quiet time alone with Him. Get to know Jesus personally, getting fully cooked in the Lord so you will be popped to perfection when He comes to take you home.

When things come into your life and try to stop your cooking time, just remember the scriptures and promises you have in Christ. Fight back with your favorite verses hidden in your heart. Four of my favorite scriptures are Galatians 2:20 (I have been crucified with Christ...gave Himself for me), Romans 8:28 (All thing work together...for Gods purpose). Philippians 4:13 (I can do all things... Christ's strength) and Acts 20:24 (But my life is worth nothing unless I use it for doing the work...by the Lord Jesus...kindness and love). When your heart is popped to God's perfection, you will have faith hidden deep inside your heart that the Holy Spirit will bring to your remembrance when you need it. So make sure there are no hidden husks left inside your heart. Confess your sins, study your Bible, and build your prayer life with Jesus and fellowship with other believers.

Just as a fluffy white piece of popcorn can be popped to perfection when it is fully cooked, you too will have a fluffy pure heart filled with God's love, His Word and His promises as you draw near to Him on a daily basis. Jesus will one day bring to light the hidden things of darkness (Ecclesiastes 12:14 and I Corinthians 4:5). So get those hidden things cleaned out now while you have the opportunity to do it.

Let us pray:

Lord I lift my heart up to you and ask your forgiveness from the known and unknown sins in my life. Pop my heart to your perfection, Lord, fluffy and pure by the Blood of Christ. Take out all my hidden sin that hides in the deep, dark, places of my heart. Pour out your Holy Spirit, Father, and open my heart so I can be open to your presence, ready to receive the things from you that you have for me to do. Let me be a willing vessel and serve you Lord. I repent from my sins *(name them if you know which ones the Holy Spirit is showing you)* and I receive, by faith, the Blood of Christ over them, in Jesus' name I pray. Thank you Lord, for the blood you shed on the Cross for ALL my sins. Thank you, Lord, for the Holy Spirit who leads me into all truth and helps me to understand the things you are saying to me about my heart. Thank you, Lord, that you will show me the hidden junk in the dark places of my heart so I can repent and be cleansed as you make me whole again in you.

Thank you, Lord Jesus, for the promise of eternal life with you in Heaven. Thank you, Jesus, that in you, there is no condemnation and I am forgiven because of God's grace and mercy. Thank you, Father God that I can confess my sins and you are faithful to forgive and cleanse me. To Jesus I give all the praise, for He alone is worthy to receive ALL glory. In Jesus' name I pray. Amen.

Written By: Thelma Conway
4 November 1964

I Make a Stand

Deep down in my heart is a spot
I keep under lock and key –
Although it is a very small slot,
I shall always remember thee!

Old memories keep coming back
And though at times they haunt me –
The world at times looks very black
What are these things we cannot see?

Oh, Lord above – be my helpful one
To cast away all stones and sand
Come down from Your Heaven up above
Help me, please, to make my stand!

I stand on firm ground for all to see
The world revolves on and on
Oh, dear Lord, I cling to thee
Before another day has gone.

My children are all growing so fast –
I fear I may lose them now,
The Lord, I see has come at last - -
To help, for I cannot, somehow!

He helps us, though we do not see - -
But in our heart we know Him
If we believe, forever we will be
Closer to Him, we will show Him

I love Him, with all my heart, my mind
I know that He believes me - -
Forever the light in His eyes will shine
So all of us can see THEE!

Strength in the Lord

Tonight as I sat down to polish my nails and the thoughts from the day were on my mind, there was such a peace in my spirit about my relationship with the Lord. It was a feeling I had felt before when I received Jesus as my personal Savior and I was born again *(John 3:3 and John 3:7)*. The peace I felt back then came over me again. It was just as strong now as it was the first time. That feeling of freedom in my spirit and the burdens being lifted off my shoulders felt so peaceful and calming to my soul tonight. As I sat on the porch, doing my nails God began speaking to me about many things taking place in my front yard. I was watching my grandchildren (Chase, Little James and Matthew) play football with both my daughters' (Crystal and Angel) boyfriends (James and Stacey, who are now their husbands). All of a sudden, Crystal and Angel jumped in the game to help Chase, Little James, and Matthew win the game against Stacey and James. Our two dogs (Prince and Pooh Bear) were playing all around them and would not listen to what the kids were telling them to do. The dogs were getting in the way and messing up their great football game. Even with all the commotion and arguing back and forth between them, you still could see the love they had for each other. As I watched everyone playing, I felt such love in my heart. It felt like heaven had opened up and God was pouring His love out as He showed me how much He loves us, even when we are arguing and playing. He loves us unconditionally with a heart that is pure love. God always pours His love in us but most of the time we do not recognize it when we are doing our own thing. I am learning to look at His love more and more every day when I go into my secret place with Him and talk about everything.

Tonight I was excited to hear what the Lord wanted to share with me. As I was putting on my nail polish, which is a nail hardener and strengthener, God gave me a wonderful revelation about the strength in the Lord *(Philippians 4:13)* and how everything I do I can do with His strength. Just as the polish strengthens my nails, I am strengthened in Him.

The nail polish I was using has fibers in it and when you apply two coats, it makes your nails stronger. My nails are weak and I needed the fibers to give them extra strength so they would not break. God spoke to me and said, "Randy, as the fibers in the polish are making your nails stronger, your faith in the Cross of Christ makes your spirit stronger." As I was putting on the polish, I could already see how strong my nails were becoming. Now, I can understand how the Blood of Jesus, that covers our sins, make our spirit stronger. We have been set free and there is no longer any guilt or shame in Christ Jesus. At that moment, I saw a vision of Jesus' Blood flowing over my whole body and all my sins were being washed away. I am clean, forgiven, and reconciled back to God by Christ's Blood *(Romans 3:21-26 and Romans 5:8-11)*. After I put the red colored polish over the nail strengthener, I could not see the ugly fibers on my nails any longer because the fresh, clean, shiny red polish now covers them. I believe God does not see our sins any longer because of the Blood of Christ that covers them. I sat there overwhelmed by the grace and mercy God has given us through Jesus and wondered why some people just do not want to know Him. When you share the word with some people they may say, "I am not interested," or they may say, "I don't want to hear about God because there are too many hypocrites in the church and if that's what it's all about I don't want it." As the red polish covered my ugly nails with its shiny new color, Christians need to let the Blood of Christ cover our sins, showing God's love and the character of Jesus. If people could just experience God's love and get to know Him, they would never be the same again!

As I sat there, I thought about putting on another coat of shiny red polish, wondering if I really wanted to. I did not want to wait for the first coat to finish drying because I was in a hurry. If I put another coat on my nails too soon it would mess up the smooth look I now have. I knew I had to put another coat on if I wanted them to be stronger, so I waited to put the second coat on.

Every day we need to apply the Blood of Christ to our lives and put on the full armor of God, walking with the Holy Spirit daily *(Ephesians 6:10-20)*. You see, many walk around in the world with one coat of Jesus' Blood on them. They think because they accepted Christ once that is all they have to do. We need to apply the Blood of Jesus and die daily (confess our sins as Paul teaches us in the Word of God). Do not be impatient, but wait for God to reveal all your sins to you. When we wait on God we get cleansed and then we can stand against the evil in the world. Sometimes we think we have confessed everything and are finished, covered by the Blood, and we leave until the next time we need forgiveness. The Holy Spirit convicts us *(John 16:8)*, of sin so we can repent and be covered with a fresh coat of Christ's Blood. We need to wait in God's presence until He is finished with us. We cry out to God for help in confessing, but we sometimes do not wait for the Holy Spirit to finish with us because we are in a hurry. We may still be wet and need another coat of Christ's Blood over an unconfessed area in our lives.

We walk away wet until the next time we mess up and confess that present sin. We need to take time to wait in the presence of the Lord to get completely dry, convicted of the sins that the Holy Spirit wants to reveal to us. We are putting Christ's Blood over the present sin and hiding the ugliness, but each time we sin, we forget that there may be those things hidden inside us, like bitterness, anger, gossip or some unforgiveness. God wants to cleanse our heart of everything that is not of Him. We will get that smooth, fresh, shiny coat of Christ's Blood and continue on with smiles on our faces, but we will not be still long enough to hear the Holy Spirit telling us, "There is something else I want to talk to you about. Let's take care of this sin too." We may think we are getting stronger in our walk, but we are not getting as strong as God wants us to be with the deeper truth of salvation through the convictions of the Holy Spirit. Yes, we are saved by grace in faith because of Christ, and not by religion and the law *(Galatians 2:16-21)*. We are fully trusting in God's promises for heaven and believe in faith *(Galatians 3:5-14)* but God wants a closer, intimate relationship of love with us as He draws us nearer to Him by His Holy Spirit.

Weakness in our flesh is a good thing, for to be weak in our flesh, we are strong in Christ. The revelation is that the weakness is a thorn in our flesh and reminds us of our need for God *(II Corinthians 12:7-10)*, because God is all we need. Having strong nails with the polish and strengthener is like having strong minds with the word of God through the polishing of the Holy Spirit's teachings. We must also remember not to let Satan deceive us with his lies, but forgive everyone so we can be forgiven. To do this we stop Satan with the word of God *(II Corinthians 2:10-11)*. Satan will try to encourage us to keep those hidden sins. The Holy Spirit will convict us of our sins so we can repent. We need to wait in the presence of God each time we go before Him and confess everything.

God's Word says all we need to do is have faith in the Cross of Jesus, His death and resurrection, that He is the **ONLY** Son of the living God, believing with our whole heart all the promises in the Bible and we will be saved and have eternal life with Him forever. If we do not believe Jesus really died for us, we are really not trusting God. We have to take captive the lies of the enemy with the Word of God and what the Holy Spirit is revealing to us. God loves us so much and wants us to see how very important it is to keep our eyes on Jesus and be open to the convictions of the Holy Spirit, so we can have a pure heart. We draw strength from the Lord as the Holy Spirit teaches us all things. Peace fills our soul as we sit in the presence of God waiting on Him to speak to our spirits.

I encourage you all to be open to whatever God wants to tell you. Believe, in faith, that it is the Holy Spirit unveiling those hidden sins inside you, so that the Blood of Christ can be freshly applied to your heart each day of your life. Just as a lady's nail polish can wear off her nails and she might need a fresh coat to make them look shiny again, our hearts need to be freshly polished each time we sin with a fresh coat of the Blood of Christ. It is not that the Blood of Christ will ever wear off, but it needs to be freshly applied each day for protection in our hearts as the shiny polish protects our nails. We do not know when Jesus is coming back for us so we need to be ready at all times.

Let us pray:

Father, we thank you for the Blood of Christ and give you praise for the convictions of the Holy Spirit. Lord, without you we would not have the Holy Spirit. It is because of your sacrifice on the Cross that we are saved. Lord, help us to be more patient and wait in your presence to hear your voice inside us telling us the things we need to confess so that we will have a clean pure heart before you each day. Give us strength to fight the enemy and stand on your word of truth that you have given us. Help us to remember that each day we need to apply a fresh coat of the Blood of Christ and put on the full armor of your Word so we can walk on the narrow path to your holiness. Thank you, Father, for your grace and mercy. Thank you, Lord God, for your love that pours out on us daily by your Holy Spirit. Thank you Lord, for the peace you pour into our spirits with your presence. It is in Jesus' name we pray.

Written By: Thelma Conway
5 November 1964

Trusting In Him

Our Lord above has staked His claim –
Each one in life has a definite aim
A time to be born, and a time to die - - -
Before he reaches that heaven on high.

We will be patient, though hard it must be
We live on land, underground, on the sea –
Each day a different challenge comes into view
It's up to each of us to know what to do!

We go about, normal to what is around
Though at times our lives may go aground –
We believe in God, our trust is in Him
Although at times, the light does grow dim!

Hold your head up high for all to see –
When in the dumps, God will rescue thee
Start each new day with a new beginning
Wake up each morning with a bit of singing.

Speak to God each day, the Bible you must read
Speak the Words from His Book, and then take heed
A verse a day will give you new hope
You will never again sit around and mope.

Give of yourself, give till it hurts
You know each day what you have to do.
Give of yourself – use your heart some
And you will find, "God to you will come!"

I say hurry on – the day is young still
Deep in your heart you have the will
Go on living in your own way
And remember: "Speak with God" every day!

A Christian's Teddy Bear

(This story is dedicated to Angel)

It was 5 March 1997, early afternoon and a rather quiet day at the office. While having a conversation with a co-worker, I listened as she shared a story with me about a teddy bear her dad had given to her when she was a little girl. The Holy Spirit quickly brought to my attention how parents can lead their small children to the Lord. Children trust their parents for everything. The Holy Spirit revealed to me it is not just about leading our children to the Lord, but about leading any child, teenager, or grown adult to Jesus. The Lord says He is the vine and we are His branches *(John 15:5)*. It is up to us to tell people about Jesus, plant the seed, and allow the Holy Spirit to draw them to Jesus for salvation.

As I thought about my co-worker's story, it took me back to my own experience with a teddy bear Allen (my husband) and I had given to our youngest daughter, Angel. She was thirteen days old at the time, sick in the hospital and in isolation with a staph infection. Her Dad brought a cute brown teddy bear for her and wanted Angel to love it as much as he did. He wanted to make the teddy bear special to her. Angel was so tiny lying in that big hospital bed and because she was in isolation, we were not allowed to take the teddy bear in the room, so it had to stay out on the cart by her door. Day after day as I sat in the room with her, I looked at that teddy bear and wanted so badly for our little girl to have him. It meant so much to Allen and me, but our baby girl did not even know it existed. As time went on, Angel got better; we were able to take that teddy bear in the room. When we brought her home from the hospital, we began to make the teddy bear become special to Angel. We would constantly try to make that bear a part of her by taking it everywhere she went, or making her sleep with it, and putting it on the table while we ate. For years, we tried very hard to make the teddy bear become part of her very soul because we loved it so much and wanted her to love it as much as we did. As Angel grew older, she learned to love that teddy bear on her own. In time, it meant something special to her too, and we no longer had to do anything to make the teddy bear part of her heart. She made it become part of her own heart when she fell in love with it for herself, because of the time she spent with it.

Philippians 4:13 says we can do anything with the strength of Christ. As we read God's word, pray, spend personal time alone with Him and worship with other believers, God starts to become part of our soul. The Holy Spirit will fill us with Jesus as we seek His presence. The more we spend time with God in His Word the more we will grow and become a part of the branch on God's vine. We will grow and blossom as we focus on Jesus and listen for His voice speaking inside us. God will grow in us daily as we do our personal devotions with Him one on one. Eventually one day we will be grown and matured in the Lord and can lead others to the Lord so the Holy Spirit can draw them into salvation. Our roots will become part of a vine rooted in Christ because He first loved us *(1 John 4:19)*. Being a part of God's vine, our branch will hold His fruit for others to see Him in us, and they will begin to hunger and thirst and want to eat of the same fruit we have. People will become filled with the fruits of Jesus and be a branch on God's eternal vine.

Christians must continue steadfast in their walk with Jesus, focusing on Him and seeking His face for everything in their lives. The only way we become rooted in Christ is by staying in fellowship with other believers and building a daily personal relationship with God in His Word and in prayer. We must make Jesus part of everything we do, just as we made the teddy bear part of every thing Angel did. If we do not stay in fellowship with Jesus and read the Bible, we will not grow and we will fall off the vine of life. Being with other believers, we can encourage one another in Christ, and we will eventually begin to grow in our relationship with Him all on our own. As we continue to grow, never giving up, we will not have to be taught to love Jesus, or to love one another. It will just happen and it will become a part of our everyday life because we are in love with God. We will love because Jesus is part of our very soul and we will be planted and rooted in Christ's love.

The fruit will blossom as we share God's Word and show others by our actions and character. As unbelievers watch our lives and start seeing how we show Jesus in us by the things we do, how we act, and what we say, they will become even hungrier to be part of God's vine and they will want to be rooted in Him too. "Greater is He who is in me…" *(1 John 4:4)* is what the unbelievers will see in our character. They will start growing up in the Lord and begin sharing the gospel on their own without our help. Jesus will work with them to spread the word of life to the unsaved. Many more lives will know Jesus as we do what He tells us to do, go into all the nations *(Mark 16:15)* and share the gospel.

We cannot keep the gospel for ourselves and not share the truth. Be obedient to what God says and share your experiences, your trials, and your testimonies. Show others how you walk with Jesus on a daily basis and how His love took you from a lost life of sin and death and gave you a promise of an eternal peace with Him. Let the Holy Spirit introduce you to forgiveness and peace in the Lord Jesus Christ who died for all mankind.

As you seek first the kingdom of God each day and make Jesus part of your daily life you will grow closer and stronger in Him and Jesus will become your own personal teddy bear. You will not want to be without Him anytime. You will take Him with you everywhere you go.

Jesus, He is a Christian's teddy bear! Make Him your teddy bear today.

Let us pray:

Lord, I thank you for your love. I thank you for my personal relationship with you. I come to you today and seek a renewing and a refreshing in my relationship with you. Fill me, Holy Spirit, with a heart like Jesus so that I can be a vessel used by God to share the gospel, His Word. Make Him my lifeline to eternity. Fill me with the power and the presence of the Holy Spirit. Take my flesh and get it out of the way so my spirit will rise and others will see that Jesus in me is greater than any other thing in my life. I want to walk and shine as a light in this world. I give all the glory, honor, and praise to Jesus, my Savior, for He is the only one who is worthy. Thank you, Jesus, for salvation. Thank you for renewing and refreshing me in my relationship with the Father, the Son, and the Holy Ghost. To God be the glory for all He has done, is doing, and will continue to do in me for His purpose. I pray in the name of Jesus.

Written By: Thelma Conway
18 October 1981

What Jesus Had Done in My Life

Oh, Jesus, let me truthfully say
I'm glad You came to me to stay
To keep me straight, to guide my ways
To be by my side now and always.

I know at times I walk a dark path alone
But always in my heart Your light has shone.
To light the way when I'm blue and sad
And let me know I'm really not all bad.

Dear Jesus, I try hard every day – You know
To do Your will like You would have me – so
Thank You, Lord, through the study, I have won
And I know now, You are the Greatest One!

The One who stands by me when I slip and fall
And catches me and makes me stand so tall
I am not ashamed for things I have done or said
Because now I am learning to live better instead.

I am so proud I am a Christian, you see
It is hard yes, but I still try to be me
I will wait upon the Lord and I will not tire
And Jesus will fill me with His fire

For there are other works that will transpire.

I shall from this time forth, soar high as the sky
Overcoming those obstacles, out the window they will fly - -
My faith and trust in You grows so very deep
I conquer my ills – even when I am asleep!

May I walk straight, love those who hate me
For this study opened my eyes and now I see
The Lord will take care of evil ones, I know
And inside now, I have the special glow.

Knowing I walk with Jesus from now on
My eyes soar like eagles and go beyond
The clouds way up high and out-of-sight

Thank you again, Dear Jesus - - I have seen the LIGHT!

Our Locked and Caged Heart

It was Friday, the morning of April 1997. I was getting ready to leave the house for work and I had put our younger dog (Pooh Bear) outside in his pen while I let the older dog (Prince) stay in the house. I stood watching both dogs staring at each other, one looking through the glass door to the outside and the other from outside in the pen looking into the house. Prince did not make a mess. He was trained so he could be left alone in the house without supervision. Pooh Bear was still being potty trained and he chewed things that did not belong to him, so we would put him in a cage that had a padlock on it. This way if anyone came in the yard they would not be able to open the gate and let him out. God spoke and I listened as He told me about the hearts of some believers. Pooh Bear was locked in his cage; he was calm and quiet, not bothered by anything going on around him. He looked so unhappy and very sad while he was looking at me standing by the glass door with Prince. Pooh Bear was probably wondering why he was not in the house with us. It was cold outside today, but we were inside, safe and warm, while he was out there, cold and caged, not knowing how to get out of that locked pen. If only he had barked or cried, my heart being full of love for him, I would have gone to him before I left for work and given him some encouragement of how much I loved him. I guess during this time I did not feel he needed me so I did not move towards him. I just stood there watching with eyes of love and compassion waiting for him to bark for attention.

Humans sometimes act like Pooh Bear, caged, locked up, and not knowing how to get out. Many do not really think they can get out. Satan has some of us locked in a cage with no way out. Some cages

41

have the latch up on the door and the door is ajar, but we do not move because we will not cry out for God's help or we may think we cannot get out. Some of us are locked up with only the latch down on the gate and it does not even have a padlock on it. We do not know how to lift the latch up to open the gate and escape. There are those who have locks on their heart with no way for God to get in at all. They are just sitting in Satan's cage thinking there is no way out of the mess they have gotten themselves into, or no way out of a situation they are facing because they don't ask anyone to help them. There maybe Christians surrounding us with the love of Christ in them, who will give us a word of encouragement if we open up to them and ask for help or even for some advice. We may be too wrapped up in our problems to feel the love of Christ flowing through others. How can people encourage us in the Lord so we can be set free, if we do not stop being self-centered? We become slaves to Satan and sin *(Romans 6:16-19)* trying to think of our own way to get out of those situations. We may wonder why we cannot figure it out on our own without bothering others for help. God does not want us to suffer alone. He put others around us to show us His way of escape so we will not be bound to those locked cages the devil puts us in.

Pooh Bear had a padlock on his cage so he could not get out, but I would have gone to him if I had heard him bark for attention. Some of us Christians have padlocks on our heart and do not allow God to set us free. We put up walls around our heart thinking we are protecting ourselves from getting hurt repeatedly by the same issue. We limit God's help and His power in our lives. We do not want to hear about God and His help because we cannot see or understand how He can help us as we look at our problems with our natural eyes. We are not showing any faith in God and we have allowed our heart to be hardened towards Him. The love of God cannot get in to bring us peace or joy. Jesus is able to unlock the cages of our heart if we will just seek the kingdom of God first and allow the walls to come down by trusting God with what we say we believe. When we share a word of encouragement or we are invited to church and listen to the message the pastor speaks, we can be set free by the truth *(Psalms 95:2-11)*. Let us come into the Lord's presence and enter into His rest worshiping our King. Jesus will close the door to Satan and throw away the locks the enemy had on our lives, if we will just cry out and ask for help.

As we keep our eyes on Jesus and the promises in God's Word, we will not be put in a cage and locked up. However, when we take our eyes off Jesus the devil can step in and mess with our heart and our mind. Do not look back at the world; keep your eyes forward on Jesus. Keep your faith locked into who you are in Him. Jesus will close those doors against the enemy, lock them with His Blood, and we will be set free. We will no longer be sad, unhappy or feel alone, out in the cold, forgotten. We will be warm, in His presence, growing in obedience to God's voice, allowing the Holy Spirit to lead, guide, and direct our lives. God tells us to be led by the spirit, not the flesh *(Galatians 5:16, 17 and Galatians 5:22-25)*. In the book of Romans, God tells us not to move in the ways of the flesh but in His spirit *(Romans 8:4)*. Jesus becomes Lord of our heart and He sits in heaven on the right hand side of God interceding for us as God gives us mercy, grace and love here on earth and then forever for all eternity.

Praise God! We have a way out of locked cages. Come to Jesus and invite Him into your heart as your Lord and Master. He is our Savior and the only way back to the Father, for He says that He is the only way *(John 14:6)* and it is through Him we must go. Jesus is the vine and we are the branches *(John 15:5)*. We can do all things through Him *(Philippians 4:13)* because He will give us strength to complete the purpose for our lives. The Holy Spirit will bring all things to our remembrance and we will have peace in our spirits. Jesus tells us not to be troubled *(John 14:26-27)*. Let us run to His arms. He is waiting to unlock those cages of our heart and mind that Satan holds captive.

I want to ask you today, what means more to you than anything else in the entire world? What would your answer be if you were asked that question? My answer is long, but to make it short, I would say, "My relationship with my Jesus"! There is nothing more than HIM that I want or need because with Him I will have everything I ever need or could ever desire. Greater is He who is in you…and that is God's truth *(1 John 4:4)*. Love one another unconditionally and share the gospel, encouraging each other in the Lord. Get out of those locked cages now and open up your heart to the Holy Spirit who will lead you into all truth. You know God will send people to you but you must be open to receive what He wants to say through them. God loves us so much and He wants to unlock all those dark places and let His light in so we can see His love for us more clearly.

Please pray with me:

Father, thank you for the light in the darkness. Thank you for unlocking the cages of my heart that Satan has put me in (open up to God and tell Him what is bothering you). Thank you Lord, for your Holy Spirit who will lead me into all truth. Thank you, Lord, for your grace and mercy. Father, I want the cages of my heart that are locked to be unlocked, and I have faith in you that you will do it. Lord, fill me with your presence that I will have boldness to share words of encouragement with others so that they will be set free from the locked doors they sit behind. Open my spirit to receive from you, your love, so that I can share with others as you have directed me to do in your word. Lord, use me and send me to those you know are ready to be set free, speaking your truth to encourage them. Thank you, Lord, for freedom in the Blood of Christ. Thank you, Lord that you never leave us as orphans. Thank you, Lord that you are always watching and waiting with unconditional love for us to come and talk with you. Unlock our caged minds, too, Father, for the battle of the mind is great, but you, oh God, are greater. Open our ears to hear clearly the Holy Spirit that we can be led by the spirit and not by the flesh. Thank you, Father! In Jesus' name we pray.

Randy B. Brown

Written By: Thelma Conway
4 September 1983

Do You Know Jesus, Too?

found it difficult today
To do what I wanted to do
Jesus said, "Do it My Way"
"And, I will carry you through!"

So, I looked up to the One Above
For I knew He was always right
I am constantly showered with His Love
As He carries me through each night.

Thank You, Lord Jesus, for caring for me
Just a humble servant of Yours now
I love You so, I want the world to see
With You – we can get by somehow.

I have inner peace and am stronger this time
Thank You again, Jesus, for being there
Now I know Your Light will always shine
And for me – You will Always Care!

(Call on Jesus anytime, anywhere, and He will hear you!)

The Rug

(This Story is Dedicated to Rob)

It was finally Saturday and the weekend was here. I woke up this morning in a great mood and could not wait to be alone with the Lord just to sit in His presence and love on Him. We talk together when I do my morning devotions. Today my husband Allen was still asleep so I sat on the living room floor and got comfortable so I could focus. We were having brand new carpet put down and I had to sit on the floor because all the furniture was on the porch and in the garage. As I picked up my Bible I asked God, "What do you want to talk to me about today, Lord?" He led me to read ***Isaiah 59:1 and I John 1:9***. The Lord says He saves and He hears when we call on Him. If we confess our sins He is faithful to cleanse us from those sins we have just talked to Him about. The Holy Spirit then directed my eyes to look at the rug all around me and asked me to look how it was covered with dirt and little carpet shavings from the past few days. Than I had a vision of our souls full of sin from the day-to-day dirt, we put in them by the things we do or say when we make the wrong choices out of the will of God. I watched as the blood flowed down my whole body just washing away all the sin and than I saw a fresh red shine in my soul. When we confess our sins that is just what Jesus' Blood does for us. It cleanses us from sin and God sees Jesus' wonderful fresh Blood and not our sins. What a wonderful vision! Even more, it was a wonderful feeling inside my heart to know I am once again washed clean from sin.

I sat there waiting to hear what God wanted to tell me about the dirt on the rug and the vision and I heard Him tell me things about the dirt in our life from day to day that needs to be cleansed with a fresh coat of the Blood of the Lamb. When we move into a new house, we clean everything before we move furniture and our other things into it. It is spotless, clean, and ready for our house to become our home. When we buy new carpet, we have to do the same thing when the job is finished. We have to vacuum and get it ready for our furnishings to be put back in place. The rug looks and feels fresh and clean the first time as we begin to live in our new environment. Our souls are like this. The first time we come to Jesus for salvation we are full of sin. Because of Adam and Eve's disobedience to God, we were born sinners. When we confess our sins to God, we receive Jesus as our Lord and Master. Jesus pours His Blood out on all our sins and they are now covered *(Revelations 1:5)*. We are fresh and clean for the first time in our life from all our sins. When we stand before God, because we are now saved and have faith in the Blood of Christ, we are free, fresh and clean in the Lord Jesus Christ, the only Son of God *(John 3:18)*. God says that old things are passed away and all things become new. He makes us new *(II Corinthians 5:7 and Revelations 21:5)*. We have become a new creature in Christ.

As time goes on, day after day, the rug gets dirty all over again with new dirt that is tracked on it. The old dirt we cleaned last week is gone. It will never be seen again and we will not even remember what it was. However, there is new dirt that comes on the rug each day that covers it and we need to clean it up again. We will pull out the vacuum, suck up all that new dirt so it is fresh, and clean once again to be presented to our company as something spotless.

Our souls can be cleaned just like the rug is cleaned everyday. Each time we mess up and slip away from the will of God, back into the world, we can come to God and repent. We will be cleaned again fresh and new in Him and He says that He will forgive us and remember our sins no more *(Jeremiah 31:34c)*. When we first came to Jesus for salvation we received His Blood covering for our sins and then the Holy Spirit came in us and sealed us in the arms of God *(Ephesians 1:13)*. Jesus is in heaven on the right hand of God but He left us the Holy Spirit to guide and teach us. The Holy Spirit will bring things to our attention and tug at our heart when we sin so we can be quick to repent and seek forgiveness and be cleansed by the Blood of Christ again for a fresh new covering of the Blood of the Lamb. The Bible teaches us to die daily *(I Corinthians 15:31)*. As we are, open to the voice of the Lord the Holy Spirit will continue to tug at our heart cleansing us each time we sin. We will have a pure heart when we humble ourselves before God seeking forgiveness, repenting and than we are presented to the world as a Christian, trusting and believing in God for the Blood of Christ and the remission of our sins. When we die, Jesus will present us to the Father as righteous because of our faith in Him and His resurrection. The Blood of Christ will blot out our sins never more to be remembered *(Hebrews 10:15-18)* just as the rugs old dirt is never seen or remembered again.

Even though the dirt on the rug keeps coming back, and we can clean it each time, we can come to God every time we sin, repent, and be cleansed again. The rug is repeatedly vacuumed and our souls continue to be cleansed by the Blood of the Lamb as we repent daily. God forgives us because of our faith in Jesus. It is important for us to walk in the light of Christ with the Holy Spirit leading us and confess our sins, dying daily as Paul teaches us to do. Jesus will be glorified as we give Him the honor, praise, and thanks for all He has done for us. He freely gave His life for our sins. There is no cost to us for salvation. All we have to do is go before the Throne of God and repent (turn away from those sins) and receive by faith what

Jesus did for us on the Cross (He was crucified, dead and buried and in 3 days He rose from the dead and He is the ONLY BEGOTTEN SON OF GOD).

We become clean, fresh and new daily as the rug does each time it is vacuumed. When we keep our eyes on the Lord, put our faith and trust in Jesus, God does see our repented heart. He has cleansed us; we will have eternal life in heaven with God forever. Only Jesus can clean our heart and make it pure, fresh, and new again. We are in Christ now and belong to Him because we gave Him our life that moment we received Him as our Savior. We have been adopted into the family of God through the Blood of Christ.

When you are looking at your own rugs and the dirt on them remember to let the Lord speak to your own heart and reveal your sins daily as you confess before Him. Be humble at the Throne of mercy and grace and allow God to continually cleanse your repented heart. Jesus will present you before our Father in heaven as a clean and pure vessel.

Please pray with me:

Father, first we thank you for the Blood of Jesus and we thank you for the Holy Spirit. We confess our sins before you now, Lord *(name them as the Holy Spirit brings them to your remembrance),* and seek forgiveness and a fresh new covering of the Blood of Christ. Father, we repent and ask for your strength to continue pressing forward. We pray, Lord that as we die daily you will continue cleansing our heart. Father, we want to be presented before you, by Jesus, with a clean, pure heart, forgiven, and live eternally with you in heaven forever. Thank you for your promises and your faithfulness. We thank you that you do not remember our sins once we have repented and that we are free, fresh and new in the spirit. Help us not to go backward but to keep pressing forward. Keep us clean and present us to the world as your children, saved by the Blood of the Lamb. Open our ears so we can clearly hear the Holy Spirit showing us our sins and we can confess all of them. Open our heart to receive your presence as we stand before your Throne. Thank you, Jesus, for reconciling us back to the Father. Thank you, Jesus, for not giving up on us. To you, Lord, we give all the glory, honor, and praise and we pray in your holy and righteous name.

Randy B. Brown

Written By: Thelma Conway
4 September 1983

Let Me Walk With You

Jesus, let me walk with You
Jesus, let me take Your Hand
Because I know You Understand –
And, You are Always There!

Please – help me keep You Near
Always I will look to Thee
I know You will stay beside me –
You are with me everywhere!

(Cast your burden upon the Lord – Psalm 55:22)

The Old Chocolate Candy Bar

(This story is dedicated to Crystal)

I felt discouraged again this morning as I got out of bed. For the last few days I had been depressed and having a hard time functioning with all these thoughts going through my head. Today was only Wednesday in the month of November of 1999. I knew I had a lot to get done at work today but I was still worrying about our oldest daughter, Crystal, and my mind was just not thinking about work. A few days ago she found out she was having her second child and I was concerned about their finances. Wondering how she and her husband would be able to afford two children, I went on to work again still depressed. I was having a hard time concentrating on anything I did. All I could do was think about Crystal and her family. I was happy they were having their second baby but I was too busy condemning myself for the way I was feeling about my daughter. In the past few days, I have not been able to hear the Lord's voice speaking to me. I did not even take time to stop long enough to listen if He had tried to get my attention. I was to busy figuring things out for them myself. Later on in the early part of the afternoon, sitting at my desk, my mind had quieted down and I was able to get some work done. Finally, it was quiet in my head! As I concentrated on work again, I heard God's voice softly calling my name. I listened to His voice inside me and realized I should have gone to Him long before this! Sometimes we are so wrapped up in our own thoughts we do not ask God for help. We think our problems are something we can take care of and will not bother God with this one. The Lord spoke my name again just as softly as He had before and I knew He wanted my attention. "Yes, Lord," I said. God spoke I listened. He said, "Randy, remember how you felt when you found out Crystal was coming?" "Yes Lord, I do", was my response.

Crystal was our second child. On the day I found out she was coming to join our family of three, Allen, and I were having a hard time with finances and in our marriage. Although things were not the best for us, God was at work with His mighty hand of mercy on the baby who was growing inside me. He knew this child had a lot to give to the world. He created her for His purpose and He used us to be her parents. God was blessing the baby I was carrying and it was up to Allen and me to make the choice to have her. See the doctor wanted me to abort her because of our situation; but we did not believe in abortion. We trusted God to take care of everything that lay ahead for us. Even though we did not think we could afford another baby, the Lord knew we could, because He would be the one providing everything we needed.

Today as I got up I was burdened with the way I felt years ago when I got pregnant with Crystal. I still, after all these years, felt guilty about those feelings I had so long ago. I thought about what the Lord has since done in her life, and how she serves Him. I began to condemn myself more and more for those old feelings. They were still deep inside my heart and I had not forgotten them. Crystal has devoted her life to God, and she is on a road of righteousness in Him. The last few days Satan had been reminding me of what I felt years ago when I found out our second child was coming and he filled my head with so much guilt, I could not even eat or collect my thoughts. I was overwhelmed with grief and anger at myself for those feelings. I began to question my salvation and wondered how God could still love me when I did not want to have my baby. Even though it was so many years ago, the memory still haunted me. I love Crystal so much. I have been blessed to be her mother and she has a wonderful spirit of the Lord within her that carries the character of Christ. Jesus said we are not condemned when we are in Christ (**Romans 8:1**) so why was I letting the enemy haunt me like this? Praise God for this wonderful word the Holy Spirit brought to my remembrance. God's timing for every situation in my life has been perfect. I had been so busy figuring things out for myself and condemning myself that I could not hear the Holy Spirit trying to remind me of that scripture. I have wasted days in depression when all I had to do was stop and cry out to the Lord and listen.

Our church was having prayer in the mornings during this time so I decided I needed to get there this morning. I asked the ladies to pray for Crystal and me. They all knew what God has done in Crystal's life, and they see what her life has become. I am proud that she is my daughter. I am thankful to God for guiding Allen and me with the decision not to abort her due to our temporary lack of worldly things. Walking with God or not, your spirit knows that God's choice is LIFE, not death. Even though at that time in our lives neither Allen nor I were in a relationship with the Lord, we still knew enough about God to make the right choice about abortion. We became the proud parents of three children: Robert Allen, our oldest child; Crystal Denise, our second child; and Angela Rachel, our last-born.

I was so blessed the day we had Crystal. When she was born, she was so beautiful. She had lots of thick black hair and she looked like a little angel. I remember looking at her in my arms the morning of her birth, and crying all afternoon because I could not believe I ever felt I could not afford this little baby God put in my hands to take care of. I have repented over and over so many times for those feelings. Every time I would pick her up, I would cry out to God for forgiveness. I did not know God then the way I know Him today, and I did not understand that I only had to ask Him one time in the name of Jesus, and He would forgive me.

These were just some of the thoughts going through my mind the last couple of days. Why were these thoughts on my mind now? That was so long ago, and I was forgiven. Since developing my relationship with the Lord over the last four years I knew better than let my past sins bother me. I now know what was happening to my head; it was the enemy and not I at all. I believe I never forgave myself when I asked God to forgive me so the enemy was able to get through that open door in my life and mess with my past mistakes. You see, Satan has a way of reminding us of our past and making us feel guilty for the things we did, even when we have been forgiven of those sins. Satan has fun playing with our minds, because that takes our focus off the Cross. When we trust in God, He makes a way for us even though we see it as impossible. All things are possible in Him (**Matthew 19:26**). God made a way for Allen and me years ago when we had our second child so I know He will make a way for Crystal's second child too.

As I sat at my desk getting more depressed with condemnation, I finally decided it was time to get out of the office and renew my mind now that I know the truth. I walked down the hallway to get some coffee, and noticed that someone had put a rather large chocolate candy bar on the table for everyone to enjoy. I opened it up and saw that the candy bar was very old. When chocolate is old, it gets white spots all over it. I could see white dusty spots on the chocolate. As I looked at the candy bar, God spoke and I listened as He reminded me of how we look at ourselves. He said we see ourselves in that sinful way before we are saved. We see what we looked like before Christ and not how we look now after we are saved. We do not see what God sees, that we are in Christ, covered by the Blood. We look with our human eyes and cannot understand the beauty God sees through the Blood of Christ. Even though Jesus has changed us, we continue to look at the old ugly self we once were. God told me that He sees the change within our new heart. He sees the Blood of His Son when He looks at us now. God is molding us and making us into the image of His Son because we are born again through the Blood of the Lamb. It was at that point I realized the truth: we all need to stop looking at the world through our own eyes and learn to look at our new heart through the eyes of God. I know we cannot see through God's eyes literally, but we know now that he sees us through "rose colored glasses". The rose color is the Blood of Christ that covers up the past life we once lived, before we were saved. God wants us to stop condemning ourselves (*Job 15:5-6*). Jesus does not condemn us. We need to see who we are now in Christ, and not who we once were before Christ. We no longer look like that old chocolate candy bar. We are brand new, covered by the Blood, a new person. The old is passed away, and everything now becomes new. We are changed, a new creature in Christ (*II Corinthians 5:17*). Praise God for the Blood of Jesus!

God had given me a new revelation in my heart today, using an old chocolate candy bar to illustrate how He sees my heart now. I felt wonderful! The depression left and I could breathe again. The Holy Spirit brought so much comfort and peace to my mind; I was able to sort things out more clearly. What I now see is not the old self of yesterday, but the new me, today, in Christ. I may have felt bad, felt old and ugly, felt guilty, but these were not my true thoughts. They were things Satan wanted me to feel and think about myself so

I would not be focused on who I am now. He tries to pull us away from God. The devil is the father of lies (*John 8:44*). We need to take captive *(II Corinthians 10:3-5)* those thoughts and rebuke them right away and bring every thought back in obedience to Christ.

Even though the candy bar looked old and ugly I still took a piece of it. As ugly as it was, it tasted great. I believe that because of the Blood Jesus shed for us on the Cross, we do not look ugly to God either. What Jesus sees in us is good to Him; just like that candy bar was good to my taste buds. If we stop looking back at the old, and look forward and see the new, we will see the sweetness in the Blood of Christ that fills us now. God tests the heart *(Proverbs 17:3)* and sees the sweetness inside. We are not what the world thinks we are, when it sees us on the outside. We look at each other with human eyes and think we know everything. If our heart is right with God, we can hear the voice of the Holy Spirit and He will reveal all the truth to us. When Satan lies to us, we will be able to stand up against him and fight back with the truth in scriptures. Our heart can be filled with the joy of the Lord as we praise and worship God during times like this, instead of dwelling on the past. We must look past our natural eyes and see through the eyes of Jesus. The way to get rid of the old and ugly thoughts is to stop looking at our flesh and look at our forgiven heart. Our heart belongs to Jesus now, not the world. Let us start looking up instead of down. Start looking inside your heart instead of looking outside at the flesh. We are not today who we were yesterday. Each day is a new day in Jesus. He loves us and we love Him. He loves who we are becoming in Him because of our faith. The old has passed away, and we are new creatures in Christ *(Romans 3:22-25)*.

The old chocolate candy bar looked ugly to my eyes today, but it tasted great and I got a great revelation from God to share with you. Now joy has filled my soul instead of the lie of depression!

I want you to know something else about our Crystal. She and her family are now in Italy working as missionaries, planting new churches for the Lord. So you see God's plans were far greater for her than I could have ever imagined they would be. She and James (her husband) now have three children blessing their home. What more could a parent want than for their children to be walking with the Lord, serving Him, and for them to have that personal relationship with Him? I praise God for Jesus and the Holy Spirit. The truth is from God. All good things come to us from His hand. I know, for I have seen it repeatedly in my own life. Even as I stop and wait in His presence, the love He pours out on me is so overwhelming at times, I do not know why these last few days I did not go to Him first. I believe it was because I knew God forgave me but I did not realize that I had not forgiven myself yet. God created the universe; He is the most High God. He is Alpha, Omega, the first, and the last. God created me and if He forgives me who did I think I was not forgiving myself? Did I really trust that the Lord forgave me? This is just one of the questions we need to ask ourselves first before we let the enemy play with our past. I have learned form this experience to seek God's truth first, before I let the enemy mess with my head. I also have learned to check myself to see if I am trusting in the Word of God when the past is haunting my mind. Do I, or do I not, believe I am forgiven? What a scary experience this chocolate candy bar has given me today. Remember, when Satan tries to bring up the past, ask yourself a few questions first before you allow the depression and condemnation set in. God says that the old has passed away, and if He does not remember them why do we keep reminding Him of it? I knew than I never want to be reminded of those haunting memories again. I am a new creature in Christ forgiven by the blood He shed on the cross for my sins. To God be the glory forever!

Let us pray:

Father, I thank you, for the revelations of the Holy Spirit. I thank you for the truth and the new creature you are creating in me because of Jesus. I thank you that you can take something like a simple candy bar and bring comfort to my broken heart. Lord I love the way you use unique things to get my attention. Father, bless me and forgive me of my sins and refresh my mind with your thoughts that are the truth. Lord, help me not to keep looking back at my past mistakes, but help me to press forward and see through your eyes who I am becoming in Jesus. Father, thank you, for each day being a new day in Jesus and because of His death on the Cross I am set free, cleansed, and forgiven from all sins when I come before your Throne of grace and mercy. Old things are passed away and you do not remember them, so please help me to take captive the lies of the enemy and recognize them before I get too deeply involved in my thoughts. Thank you, Lord, for your loving-kindness. In Jesus' name I pray.

Written By: Thelma Conway
15 March 1953

Having Faith in God

When you left me, broken-hearted and blue--
I was lost, bewildered, not knowing what to do!
My life was a shambles, simply a mess
But I had 3 children, whom heaven had blessed!

I look back now and wonder how I got by--
But you know, with God watching from the sky--
He takes care of children and folks like me
Showing us what before we could not see.

I thank God! For in Him is my faith, my trust, my heart
I knew then and now know, my children from me would ne'er part!
Bless their little heart for helping me keep my head
For many was the time – I too, wanted to be dead!

God shows us the way and protects us too!
Helps us through many days that are blue --
My heart and home at last are almost one
Thanks be to God for the work He has done!

So, if you keep your head and give your heart to God,
Many the pathways and byways you will have trod!
Keep your chin up, He will make you strong,
And show you that in this world – YOU DO BELONG!

The Ice Cream Experience

Today was a Tuesday in April of 2001, in the cool of the afternoon sun, during lunch; I had gone to the store to purchase something cold and sweet. Ice cream came to my mind very quickly. What kind would I like? As I looked at all the flavors, I spotted it! Caramel Crunch ice cream! WOW!!! My eyes got big with excitement as I saw the wrapped ice cream bars in the package sitting on the shelf. I knew this was the kind of ice cream I wanted. In my mind, my eyes pictured that it would be chocolate covered vanilla ice cream bars with a crunchy rice crispy cereal and a creamy caramel filling inside the vanilla ice cream bar. The Caramel Crunch ice cream sounded good to my mind and I knew when it hit my mouth I would be satisfied with what I had chosen. While I was paying for it at the register, my mouth watered for the taste of this wonderful vision I had implanted in my mind. I could hardly wait to get back to the office to eat it. To the car I went, with anticipation of unwrapping this lovely vision of that ice cream.

Driving back to the office my head was filled with what I thought that ice cream was going to taste like and what I expected it to look like when I opened the wrapper. When I got in the office, I struggled to open the package and my mouth was watering even more. All of a sudden, my heart sunk down to my feet when I saw that the ice cream was not what I had pictured in my head. It was not chocolate covered after all. It did not have that wonderful layer of caramel filling inside it. What it did have was the vanilla ice cream bar inside a hard shell caramel colored coating. The crunch was not the rice crispy type crunch layered in the chocolate, but nuts layered over the vanilla ice cream bar. Boy was I disappointed!

As I ate the ice cream, I laid the wrapper on my desk, so I could look at the wording on it and figure out why the name of the ice cream sounded so good, but my mind pictured something else to be in the wrapper than what I was eating. The Lord began to show me my heart and the heart of many Christians. The Lord brought to my spirit *(Luke 11:39)*, the scripture about the hypocrisy of the Pharisees and lawyers. We have a face that people can see on the outside but they cannot see what is on the inside of us, what we really look like to God. People do not see the inner feelings we have. They only hear what we say, but they cannot see our mind and know how we really feel or what we are really thinking about. They do not see that our heart also have shells or walls we have put up around them, to protect us, because of past experiences from the world. We play face and word games with people.

The wrapper around the ice cream bar fooled my eyes. It was not until I opened it up and began to eat it that I saw the true picture of what was under the wrapper. As things turned out, it also tasted different from what I had anticipated too. All I had seen at first was a beautifully wrapped ice cream bar with words that drew my attention to purchase it. I had to get through the hard shell to get to the sweetness of the ice cream before I could even enjoy the fullness of the ice cream.

I believe God was showing me that we need to start breaking down the walls in our heart so that our true heart, the heart He sees, can be seen for what it reflects of Himself. We need to show His love, kindness, and mercy towards each other. God's eyes do not see what the world sees at all. We know what He sees is the truth. Even though we are of a pure heart because we belong to Jesus and He is constantly changing us, God wants us to be of pure minds also. I believe God was saying to me that it is time to look at our heart and start breaking down those walls of past pains and hurts made by the world, and let His love and mercy flow through our total being. We must let our mind and heart show the true feelings we have. Jesus told us to be angry but sin not *(Ephesians 4:26-27)*. It is okay to be angry, but at least let us learn to communicate with each other and fix problems *(Matthew 5:22-24)* instead of holding them inside to fester, or worse, putting on a false face and speaking false words we don't even really feel.

Christians belong to Jesus and they have new blood inside those old hearts. God is changing Christians into new creatures daily **(II Corinthians 5:17)**. It is time to let the Blood of Christ flow completely through us so that others may see the character of God inside us. We need to be strong because the Blood of Jesus is filling our heart everyday. Let us remove those wrappers and shells, and let the new inner heart of Jesus inside each one of us come forth to be seen for who we are in Him who has saved us from death. Give the glory to the only Son of God. God loves us inside and outside, but He knows what the inside looks like, even though the world can only see the outside and what we show them. We need to look up to Him and let Him show the world who we are today in Christ His Son.

Our heart is sweet in God's eyes because of Jesus. We need to learn to fight the devil with the word of God that says the old is passed away and we are new creatures in Christ. We must stop letting the enemy torment us with our old selves and see what God sees in us. We should also show the world our heart and the truth inside it. Let us begin to allow the Holy Spirit to tell us who we are in Christ *(Romans 8:16)*. It is time to take a stand for Jesus. Stand up, stand up for Jesus, and be God's soldiers of the Cross! Do not let the world speak badly of Christians any longer *(Romans 14:16-19)*. When we speak something out of our mouth, let it also come from our heart which has been cleansed by the Blood of Christ. Even though we made mistakes in the past, we are now new creatures in Christ because we have been forgiven. God does not remember our sins any longer. Satan does and he will keep reminding us of them so we will not grow and mature from the past mistakes we had made. That is how he will keep us in bondage to past sins. When we listen to Satan, we are reminding God of something He has already forgiven us of.

Do not let the world see the old person you use to be, but start letting them see the one who is a new creature in Christ. No longer let Satan make you put on a false face. Let Jesus tare down the walls Satan has around your heart that causes those strongholds in your new life. Let the world see the beautifully wrapped person who is in Christ, who is the new creature that God sees, wrapped in the Blood of the Lamb and be set free from the bondage of the past.

Please let us pray:

Father, thank you for showing me my true feelings, and what you see in my heart. Thank you, Lord that you give me grace and you love me on the inside and outside. Father, help me to see others the way you see them and to love them with your heart, not my heart that was shaped by my past hurts. Father, tear down the walls that surround my heart so I can be open and set free from the past pains which have me in bondage to Satan's lies. Father, help me learn how to be angry but sin not, and give me your strength to love others unconditionally. Let my heart and mouth speak what is the truth inside me because you have cleansed me by the Blood of Christ. Thank you, Father, for the Blood of your Son. Thank you, Father, for reconciling me back to you through Jesus' death on the

Cross. Thank you, Lord, for dying for my sins and making me a new creature in Christ. Thank you, Jesus, for the Holy Spirit who teaches me the truth about my heart so I can repent. What others see in me, a wrapper on the outside, let me be unwrapped showing the new creature I am now because of the Cross. In Jesus' name, I pray.

Randy B. Brown

Written By: Thelma Conway
2 May 1981

My Sweet Angel

There is a special little girl, who lives in our town,
Guess what her name is – Why, it's Angel Brown
She has brown eyes, and a lovely smiling face
Know what, no one could ever take her place!
She is sweet, adorable, impish, and loving too
I love her so much, when she is sad, I am blue
Did you know Rusty and Taffy love her a bunch
When she eats, they want to share her lunch.

Now, Angel is getting big, she is already four –
She reads, knows her name and oh, so much more.

How sweet it is when she hugs your neck and smiles
Says: "I LOVE YOU" – for that you'd walk a million miles!
How great it is to have Angel around –
I'm sure glad she came to OUR TOWN!
I love her so very much, I want her to know
When she comes to visit, I'm sad when she has to go –

I want her to come love me – this sweet Angel Brown
The Special Little Girl who has come to our town.

When Angel's near, when it rains, it is always sunny
Because she's a charmer, she's just a honey.
Everyone loves her, her brother, and her sister - -
When she's away, they say: "We sure missed her!"

She steals your heart, she steals the show
Angel, you're so sweet, I wanted you to know - -
All of us love you honey, "Little Miss Angel Brown"
Gosh, this Grandma's glad YOU CAME TO HER TOWN!

Keep sweet, stay pretty and be a good girl, too
And along life's way, everyone will always love you
Your Jesus smiles down from His Heaven, above
He lets you know how much you are loved!

Grandma loves you so much – "DEAR ANGEL BROWN"
I THANK JESUS for letting you come to our town!

A Heavenly Insurance Policy

It was Wednesday, April 1998, two days before the weekend. I knew we needed some money before we headed off on a trip. With this in mind, I went to the bank during lunchtime and ran into the bank manager, who happens to be a friend of my husband, Allen. Sam asked me if Allen had made any decisions yet about retiring. We talked for a while. I asked a few questions about retiring from the military. What Allen and I could do to ensure we make the right financial decisions before he retired. Sam had retired a few years earlier, and he knew what would be important when making those financial decisions. Allen and I were going through a class at the time that the government gives to active duty military members before they get out of the service, so they will be equipped with all sorts of essential knowledge. I had one question I wanted to ask Sam, but while talking about other things, the question slipped my mind. He began trying to guess what my question could have been. He made a few suggestions but they missed the mark. I had to stop right there and seek the Lord to bring it back to my remembrance. It was important to me, to ask that question, and I knew Sam would know exactly what to tell me. After a few minutes I quit trying to remember, what it was I felt was so important to ask him. I decided to depend on God to use Sam to tell me what God wanted me to hear. Seek first the kingdom of God *(Matthew 6:33-34)* and God will show you what you need to know!

Sam began to tell me about the military's life insurance policy for retirees. It is called the Survivors Benefit Plan (SBP). This is an insurance policy for the surviving spouse that they can live on for the rest of their lives as long as they remain single. Because I had sought the Lord for guidance in the middle of our conversation, I felt this must be what God wanted to tell me through Sam, so I listened very closely. Sam explained to me that you either take this plan out when you retire or you choose not to take it out at all. If you make up your mind to take it, the amount you choose is also very important to the surviving spouse, because you cannot change the amount once you make your decision. If you choose not to take the SBP, you cannot go back and change your mind after you have retired. It is very important to remember this while you are making your final decisions for retirement from the military. Sam told me to make sure Allen and I made the right decision and not to make a mistake and choose the wrong way. He said it was a good policy and it is a choice we can make only one time. It is a LIFE INSURANCE POLICY! If something were to happen to Allen, I would be able to live the rest of my life without any worries if we made the right decisions now. This is the way things were now in the military for retiring members.

I went back to work thinking about what we had talked about and the Lord began to speak into my spirit about the Blood of Christ being a Christian's life insurance policy for our eternal life with Him in heaven. It is a choice we must make now, while we are alive, to trust and receive in faith the Blood of Jesus as our Savior who died for all our sins. Once we die, we cannot make that decision because it would be too late. We need to make that decision while we are alive and be careful to make it NOW! The Bible says that we either accept Christ as our Savior, *(John 3:3, John 3:5-5)*, or we deny Him. Upon death, it will be too late to go back and change our mind because our spirits have either gone to heaven to be with the Lord, or to hell in eternal separation from Him. We either choose Jesus and eternal life in heaven with Him, or, we choose death for all eternity in hell *(John 3:16-17)*. It is our choice and we must not make the wrong one. We cannot risk waiting too long because we do not know how long we have. Only God knows that. He is the only one who has the power of life and death.

Christ's Blood is our HEAVENLY INSURANCE POLICY to get us to God's kingdom upon our death *(John 3:14-15)*. The Blood of Jesus insures that we are protected from death for all eternity *(Ephesians 2:13-16)*. Christ's Blood covers all our sins because He paid for them with His death on the Cross *(Matthew 26:28)*. It will cost us a decision to receive Him as our personal Savior, or it will cost us death, not receiving Him as our personal Savior. Receiving Christ's Blood atonement for our sins is the only way that reconciles us back to God *(Romans 5:9-11)*. The heavenly insurance policy is a wonderful investment into our eternal life with Christ. Make the decision now because you can NEVER go back and change your mind once you die. It will be too late.

The choice of a heavenly insurance policy must be explained to the entire world *(Luke 24:46-47)*. Time is growing very short because we do not know when Jesus is coming back to take us home. The unsaved need to make that decision now before it is too late. What better insurance policy could we have than an eternal policy of the Blood of the Lamb of God *(Hebrews 10:12-23)*? We don't even have to pay for this policy because Jesus freely laid down His life for us and He will never turn us down as long as we hold on to our faith. The rewards we get will not be cashed in on earth because God's rewards are in heaven. When we stand before God upon death and claim our sins have been bought with the heavenly insurance policy, Jesus is the one cashing in on us as He stands with us before God as our Advocate. He freely gave His life for all our sins and when we receive Him, by faith, we belong to Him for all eternity because of God's grace. No one can take us from the Father's hands *(John*

10:28-30). All we have to do is say YES to Jesus now, receive our heavenly insurance policy in faith, and know it is worth an eternal life with great rewards in heaven from God's own hand of mercy. Jesus has carved us in the palms of His hands *(Isaiah 49:15)*. Jesus will never leave us either. God will put His angels charge over us to keep us in all our ways *(Psalm 91:9-12)*. If we do not choose Jesus, we will live without Him for all eternity. An earthly insurance policy is an earthly thing worth nothing in heaven. The heavenly insurance policy is worth everything because it is eternal! The choice is ours to make NOW, while we have the chance. Come to Jesus today and repent. Be reconciled to God for all eternity. Get your heavenly insurance policy for free, which was purchased for you by the Blood of Christ, God's **ONLY BEGOTTEN SON WHO WAS THE FINAL SACRIFICE FOR ALL SIN** *(John 3:16-18)*.

Let us pray:

Father, I thank you for the Blood of Christ. I thank you that Jesus died for all my sins and I have eternal life in heaven. I believe, in faith, that Jesus is the only Son of God who freely laid down His life just for me and He bore all my sins. I thank you that you have drawn me by your Holy Spirit to Jesus. I come to you now and I invite Jesus into my heart and choose today to receive Jesus as my Lord and Savior. I receive Jesus as dying for all my sins and I repent and ask you to forgive me in Jesus' name. I believe Jesus died and rose again from the dead. I choose Jesus as my heavenly insurance policy purchased for me with His Blood on the Cross. Thank you, Lord, for saving me. Thank you, Father, that I am reconciled back to you through Christ. I ask you to fill me with your Holy Spirit who will teach me all things. Thank you, Father, for your love and your mercy through the Blood of Christ. In Jesus' name, I pray.

Written By: Thelma Conway
31 August – 1-2 September 1993

A Prayer for my Lovely Granddaughter, Crystal

My Dear Granddaughter – please know how much God loves you
He will help pull the sunshine back into a sky of blue.
If you walk "In the Garden" – and have a talk everyday
Jesus will help you, honey, "Each Step of the Way!"

When *Sally* got sick, it was something that happened that day
And Jesus looked down and said: "Crystal, I am with you all the way!"
So, put your fears aside – always rely on the Great One Above –
He will constantly wrap you forever in His arm; full of love!

Because "His Eye is on the Sparrow" – we know He loves us too
Crystal, He will help you find inner peace, so you aren't so blue!
Remember, just call on God – and talk to Him again
Because He will give you lots of sunshine – without rain.

There are lots of mountains that we all must climb –
And so much happens – good and bad – from time-to-time!
As we get down on our knees and we say our prayers
We know God and Jesus are always there and that they care!
So – we are very lucky when at times we are down - -
Friends to help, and the One who wears the Crown!

With faith the size of a mustard seed, nothing shall be impossible now
(Matthew 17:20)
For blessed be God who comforts us in all our trials, somehow
(2 Corinthians 1:3, 4)
In the world you will have troubles, but have courage, because I
have overcome the world for you
(John 16:33)
So – cast all your cares upon Him because He cares for you too
(1 Peter 5:7)

Think of all the good things that happen, the touch of Chase's cheek
And the people all around you - - who smile when you speak.
A baby can do so much to fill us full of cheer –
Every day, thank our Dear God that we have our Chase here!
And, Granddaughter, always keep your beautiful smile –
Than you will always remember, that life is so worthwhile!
Though today, it seems to you, there is so much sorrow
Things will look up; Trust in God, there will be a better tomorrow!

Because "This is My Father's World" – I know I have His love
So, totally give your heart to the Ones who live above - -
They will heal all of the feelings and your fears
And they truly are there to help wipe away your tears.

Remember, there are always better days we are told
We just have to be patient – as each day unfolds.
Know that we all love you and remember we do care
We pray for you each night, we let you know we are there!

Our Playful Puppies

It was about 9:10 in the evening, a Thursday night in June of 1997, when I was sitting on our front porch swing, like I often do when I want some quiet time alone with the Lord. Most of the time I sit alone, but for some reason tonight I let both our dogs come out with me. They alternated between playing together and growling at one another. They had no concern or worry about anything going on around them, only what they were doing right at that moment. They did not even think about the world that surrounded them, with the kids playing in the street or the cars that were passing by. As the Holy Spirit began to speak to me, while I watched these dogs, I learned from the way they were acting toward each other that they had a few human traits that were in me, and might be in you too. The human race will treat each other no different than the dogs treat each other. Just picture two puppies playing, than getting mad at each other and playing together again.

Our oldest dog, Prince, is a tiny toy mixed collie/sheltie, about 8 years old. The puppy, Pooh Bear, is a golden retriever/lab mixed, only 6 months old. When we first brought Pooh Bear home, he was just a tiny puppy, much smaller than Prince. Prince towered over him by his height and weight and pushed him around as if he were the king of the house. However, now Pooh Bear towers over Prince by much, much more, both in height and weight. He pushes Prince around now and thinks he is the king of the house. As I sat there watching them play I had to yell several times at Pooh Bear to stop hurting Prince because he was too small and getting hurt. I felt so bad for little Prince being pushed around, jumped on and pinned down by Pooh Bear. Pooh Bear was giving back some of the stuff he once received from Prince while he was smaller. The tables have turned; now, Pooh Bear is the bigger dog. I felt so bad for Prince getting hurt that I had called him to come sit by my side on the swing. I looked down at him and said, "I will protect you from Pooh Bear." All of a sudden, it dawned on me that Prince once did the very same thing to Pooh Bear. I looked down at Prince and said, "You deserve what you are getting now because you did the same thing to Pooh Bear when he was just a puppy, you reap what you sow *(Job 4:8 and Galatians 6:7)*." I said, "I love you, Prince, and I don't want Pooh Bear to hurt you. Stay here by me and I'll protect you, even though you don't deserve my protection, but I love you." Then I yelled at Pooh Bear to leave Prince alone.

The Lord opened up my heart to feel the hurt, and opened my ears to hear His voice as He began to show me things about worldly people. We go around hurting others with our mouth, our actions, or thoughts. We too deserve what we get; we reap what we have sown. God loves us too and He will protect us as we reach out and cry to Him, like I reached to Prince and drew him closer to me for protection. When we have a personal relationship with Jesus, He is there waiting to protect us because of His love for us. God covers us with peace and protection from the world. We should be focusing on Jesus and what we have in the Lord instead of what is happening around us in the world. If we do, we will react differently toward our family, friends, co-workers and other fellow men. Most of the time our feelings are our first reactions because of hurt from others. We react toward them through our feelings because of what they did or said to us. We will become offended, angry, and even bitter, and emotional, want to defend ourselves or take revenge toward others, because of the way they made us feel.

We need to start praying for them and to focus on Jesus for comfort, and ask Him to put us up on His lap and protect us from events and our own feelings. Now, there are times when we must fight back and defend ourselves so we need to ask God for discernment of the spirits *(1 Corinthians 2:10-16 and 1 John 4:1-6)*. If we will focus on the Lord, He will guide us through each battle, and give us godly reactions toward each other. The only way we will be able to hear the Holy Spirit's leading is through a personal relationship with Him. It is very important to build your relationship and keep it growing and vital, no matter what else is going on in your life. Do not give up because of what you are experiencing now. Turn your eyes to Jesus, pray, and ask the Holy Spirit to come and bring the presence of the Lord. You have not because you ask not *(James 4:2-3)*. Ask all things in the name of Jesus *(John 14:13-14 and John 15:16)*.

There is nothing more important in this entire world than our personal relationship with God. I truly believe God takes care of the world around us when we put our trust in Him. Our strength must come from God, not the world *(Philippians 4:13)*. God will use others to encourage you, too. Get into fellowship with one another and let your pastors, friends and family be your encouragers in the Lord *(Acts 2:42-44)*. We draw strength from others through the word of God, the truth. We need to start sharing what God says in the Bible. It encourages us, lifts our spirits, and will lift the spirits of others as we share. If we will look at each situation seeing things through the eyes of Jesus, He will show us how to handle it His way. God loves you so much. Our mind just cannot comprehend how much love He has for each one of us. However, we must have faith, and hope will come through faith (faith is in hearing, not seeing: **Romans 10:17**). God is always their waiting for you to ask Him for guidance. Stop seeking the world for a temporary emotional fix. Trust in God, and watch as He sends people to you from out of nowhere, simply because you have laid it all down at the feet of Jesus and asked Him for help. Pray for discernment so you will be able to recognize when God is moving. All things that come from the Father are good. God is goodness. He will turn what Satan meant for evil into something good from Jesus. If it will hurt someone, you should know it is not from God.

A personal relationship with the Lord should be NUMBER ONE in each of our lives. The only way to have that relationship is to constantly, be in the Word, in fellowship with other believers, and in prayer daily. Spend some time in fellowship with other believers. Encourage them in the Lord. Encourage someone who hurt you by planting a seed of righteousness instead of lashing back emotionally. Pray for the Holy Spirit to place a hunger in others for a personal relationship with Jesus (praying for your enemies), *(Luke 23:33-34 and Matthew 6:14-15)*. Remember, we were small once and others picked on us; but then we grew up and there are those who are smaller than us now. Instead of taking all that energy and using it to get even with someone who hurt you, use the new life you have found in Christ and spread His love and truth. Do not spread hate, anger, and bitterness. God tells us to love one another **(John 13:34)**. Share God's word. Be obedient to His commandment to love one another as He loved us.

The peace you will find in praying for your enemies is one of the most precious gifts of the Holy Spirit and it brings joy from the heart of God. Do not seek to get even, but instead spread love and peace to a lost and dying world. Time is growing shorter, my friends! We do not know how much time we have before Jesus will come back to take us home. Give everyone the same chance you have to know the truth in God's words and let them feel His love flowing through you, His vessel, and His creation. Let your love be unconditional towards one another. God loves us and commands us to love one another. He never said we would always like the way others treat us. Many did not treat Jesus with respect or love but He still loved them. So even when you are not happy with the way someone has treated you, look to God and let His love flowing through you, love them unconditionally with a Godly love. I know Jesus will take care of the emotions you are feeling inside. You will be surprised at the joy that will fill your soul because of your obedience to the word of God.

Please pray with me:

Father, I know you have given me feelings for a purpose. I ask you to show me with your Holy Spirit how to use them in a godly way and how they are to be manifested in me to bring glory and honor to Jesus. I do not want to hurt anyone any longer because of my emotional reactions to what I am feeling inside at that moment. Father, in Jesus' name, forgive me for the ones I have hurt in my life and bless them by your healing powers. Help me to focus on you first and build my personal relationship with you. I want to be used to reach out to others and encourage them with love that comes from your heart. Help me, Lord, to do as your Word says; to love one another, in Jesus' name I pray. Thank you, Jesus, for the revelations of my anger and bitterness that my emotions show towards others, so that I can repent and change. Use my emotions to glorify you. Thank you, Lord, for loving me and giving me a stronger love towards others with unconditional love, in Your Holy name I pray and thank you. Amen.

Randy B. Brown

Written By: Thelma Conway
26 March 1989 – Easter Sunday

Where Could I Go?

"WHERE COULD I GO BUT TO THE LORD" when trouble
come to me
Because "HE'S GOT THE WHOLE WORLD IN HIS HANDS"
– you see
Jesus said "FOLLOW ME" – and I will take care of you
So, "DIG A LITTLE DEEPER, IN GOD'S LOVE" and be very
true.

Because "BEYOND THE SUNSET" our parents wait patiently
In the "MANSION OVER THE HILLTOP" where everyone will be
There we will be "GATHERING FLOWERS FOR THE
MASTER'S BOUQUET"
He will give us "THE KEYS TO THE KINGDOM" that glorious
day.

And yes, "I KNOW WHO HOLDS TOMORROW" – I can plainly see
So, "FILL MY CUP, LORD" – we will be coming home to Thee!
"I ASKED THE LORD" to help me keep faith when all else fails
He said: "FAITH CAN MOVE MOUNTAINS" – you must set
your sails.

Dear God, "LET ME BE WORTHY" – of all You have done for me
Take my hand, hold fast – because "YOU BOUGHT MY SOUL
AT CALVARY"

Did you know "GOD PAINTED A PICTURE" as clear as a bell?

Go out in the world, preach His Word , all people you should tell!

"MY GOD IS REAL" – I love Him – His Son paid the price that day
He hung from the Cross that 'Black Day' and took our sins away!
So "DID YOU STOP TO PRAY THIS MORNING,"
this Glorious Easter time?
Christ rose from the dead this day, saying: "you will some
day be mine!"

And "BECAUSE HE LIVES" – oh, how great we know that song
"UNTIL WE MEET AGAIN" Lord, "LEAD ME, GUIDE ME"
– help me be ever strong
"I HAVE A PEACE IN MY HEART" because God put it there today
"ISN'T THE LOVE OF JESUS SOMETHING WONDERFUL"
– as He shows us the right way?

Pressing In

Today was our midweek service at church, Wednesday, 9 July 1997. During praise and worship, I tried hard to press into the Lord. Things kept coming to my mind about the people who were around me. I felt they were watching me and wondering how I could be so happy with all the difficulties I was struggling with. They knew the things we had been praying about for my family at that time, so nothing was hidden from them. I wondered if they thought I had a plastic face on because I was so happy worshipping the Lord in the midst of all my turmoil. There was so much going on within our family that my mind was preoccupied and made it hard for me trying to worship the Lord. I knew I needed to keep pressing into the Lord with all my heart. This was a time to let my spirit rise above my flesh. The Bible tells us to seek first the kingdom of God *(Matthew 6:33)* and that is what I truly wanted to do. The harder I tried to press in, the harder it was with all the family situations haunting my mind. The Holy Spirit stopped me in midstream as I was singing. I remember lifting my hands to the Lord to give Him my heart. As I tried harder to press in, the enemy came at me with all he had and got in my face. Right before my eyes, I saw a vision of a tall man dressed in black. He reminded me of Abraham Lincoln. He had on a tall black hat with a wide brim and he was dressed totally in black from head to foot. I had seen this man once before while I was shopping and I had gone home thinking something was wrong. However, this time he got right in my face, pointed his finger at me, and yelled in a very harsh voice. He said, "GO HOME, YOU DON'T BELONG HERE!" There was such anger in his voice I almost listened to it. I suddenly felt ashamed to worship the Lord because I knew the struggle I was having; I felt condemned. Then I remembered that Paul teaches us to press in and forget the things that are behind us *(Philippians 3:13-14)*.

It took every ounce of strength I had to stay and keep pressing in to worship the Lord. The Holy Spirit came to me and revealed to me that this man was not God telling me to go home, but it was the devil *(I John 3:20)*. I was reminded of the scripture in *1 Corinthians 12:10* where we have been given gifts of the Spirit. One of these is discernment. The Holy Spirit told me that I needed to discern the spirit that was trying to get me to leave church and know that it was not God. I knew God would never ask me to leave church nor would He condemn me. "Press into me" is what I heard in my spirit. I have to admit that at first the experience frightened me. I am thankful for the relationship I have with the Lord that I can hear the voice of God speaking in my spirit. Greater is He who is in me *(I John 4:4)*.

I stayed at church and continued pressing in during praise and worship. I knew I had just had an encounter with the enemy, but I also knew the Lord would give me strength to stand up to that ugly tall man who wanted me to leave church. As the service started, people were going up front to give their praise reports to the Lord. I knew I had one to give about my friend finding her daughter, but I even struggled with the praise report because I felt unworthy to speak it out. I told God if He wanted me to give my praise report, I needed a sign from Him. It was quiet for a few minutes and all of a sudden, my pastor asked if anyone else had a praise report to give to honor the Lord. I believed that God answered my request to Him than, so I looked at my friend and said, "I have one about my friend." She said, "Go give it." I went forward and gave my testimony.

I told the congregation that for fifteen years my friend and I had been praying for a face-to-face meeting with her daughter who had been taken from her over twenty years ago. My friend and her husband had a baby girl during a teenage relationship. Her parents gave the baby away but they told them the baby had died. She and her boyfriend were married a few years later and ended up having a son three years later. They kept trying for another baby to replace the little girl they thought they had lost, but they were never able to have one. About 15 years ago, they had found out from a family member that the first baby did not die, but was living and had been adopted by someone in the United States. Right away, my friend and I prayed for God to let her find their little girl. Finally, one day she got the news of her daughter's location. The next step was to determine how to meet with her, tell her the whole story, and initiate a relationship with their daughter. Last night my friend called me, to tell me that she finally had that meeting, and God had answered our prayers! She was so overwhelmed and encouraged because we did not give up praying. She kept her faith in God who is greater than any problem she could have. She knew God would make a way if it was His will for them to know their daughter and she said we should continue to pray until it happened.

God is so faithful! I also shared in my testimony that people need to be encouraged in their prayer life. Never give up praying for something, no matter how long it takes or even if you do not see the results. I had moved out of her state but I never quit praying for my friend. I did not talk with her on a daily basis so I never knew that she had met her daughter two weeks before she had called me that night. She did not have time to call me and tell me until then that she and her husband finally had that meeting, face-to-face, with their daughter. In the meantime, during those two weeks I still had been praying for them. God had answered our prayer two weeks earlier and my friend knew it. I had not given up praying for her. Even though you do not hear or see something with your own eyes or ears, do not give up praying until something happens. Press in to the Lord until He gives you an answer.

The Lord has given me a revelation about pressing in to Him through prayer. There are things happening in the spirit that we are unaware of when we are praying for someone. Even though my friend and I had been out of touch with each other for over a year, my prayers were still going up to the Lord for her and God was working on the answers. Pressing into God for the things of the unknown is done in faith. When the Lord reveals the answer to you, there is joy that flows through your total being that you cannot comprehend. There may be more than one level of prayer for any situation. Although the meeting had taken place, God knew my friend and her daughter still needed prayer in other areas of their relationship. There were still emotions, hurts and the pain of all the years taken from this family. Therefore, when I was praising the Lord during praise and worship I was not only concerned about my own family situation but I was also happy about my friend's situation. My face that people saw in church was not plastic at all. There was real joy in the Lord on my face, and the enemy knew it. Satan wanted me to go home because he knew if I gave that testimony on pressing into prayer, it would glorify God and defeat Satan's plan in my own life, or maybe in the life of someone else who needed to hear that testimony.

It is important to remember that God is faithful to answer your prayers, so do not stop praying even if it has been fifteen years. Great is God's faithfulness and His compassions are new every morning *(Lamentations 3:23)*. I believe God would have us encourage each other, to never stop praying for something, even if we do not know that the answer has already come. Praying builds our faith in the Lord and our personal relationship grows to new levels of intimacy with God because we are communing with Him. God will reveal the answers to us in His time. The timing is God's, not ours. Tonight was the time for me to share and encourage others about pressing into God in, prayer. I gave God the praise and honor for His faithfulness in my friend's situation, and I knew He would take care of my own situation. I needed to be faithful to my friend and pray without ceasing no matter what I was feeling emotionally in my own life.

When my pastor gave his message that night, it was all about staying in prayer, not to quit or give up because we don't see answers yet *(I Thessalonians 5:17)*. I had no idea what he was going to talk about, and he had no idea what my testimony was going to be about. As I listened to the pastor, I knew if I had listened to the enemy when he told me to leave, my testimony would not have been heard, nor would God have blessed me in what He spoke through my pastor's message. My testimony was an encouragement to others and confirmation of what my pastor preached. Through this message and the experience of answered prayer, I was so encouraged about staying in prayer. No wonder the devil came to me and tore me apart with condemnation about having a plastic face. I belonged there in church, not at home. I did press in and I am thankful the Lord gave me all the strength I needed to stand up against the enemy in that encounter!

I believe there was another message I received from this situation that night. We must go to church and be faithful in assembling ourselves together, no matter what we are experiencing in our personal life. We should not look at each other and judge people by their facial expressions. My joy was real for my friend even though I was having problems in my own life. We often judge what we see on the outside when we look at each other. We need to stop looking at each other with a judging attitude and see each other as PRESSING IN TO GOD. We may think we know all there is about someone and wonder how he or she can be so happy. We begin to judge them and think they are showing a false kind of worship. God knows our heart and He knows we are pressing in trying to focus on Him, as we should be. In addition, we all need to be in a church environment where God's presence is strong. Of course, the enemy would have us feel like we are a fake, or that we have on plastic faces. He will even try to condemn our spirits and make us want to run away. That is because the devil would have victory if we listen to his lies. However, Jesus has already won and the victory is His. There is no condemnation because we belong to Jesus *(Romans 8:1)*.

No matter what you are experiencing in your own personal life, never stop praying for others, even if you have lost touch with them. Do not stop even if you do not have any answers to your prayers yet. Praise and worship Christ and His joy will fill your soul. The joy gives you strength to fight the enemy especially while you are praising and worshiping God. Keep pressing in even when it is hard emotionally.

Please pray with me:

I praise you, Lord, and I thank you for your strength. I pray that the body of Christ will become stronger in the Lord and not get weak from worldly things. I pray that the body of Christ will unite in prayer and praise and worship you, Lord, at all times, even when we are feeling down inside our heart. I pray in Jesus' name that you, Father, would be honored with our worship, especially during the times of our pressing in when we are in the valleys, as well as when we are on top of the mountains. Help us to pray without ceasing and to remember even if we do not see your answers we should have faith that the answers are coming. For you, oh God, are faithful. All praise, no matter what we are feeling, is to bring honor and glory to you, Lord. We offer it up as our sacrifice of praise to you, for you suffered the biggest battle of all for our salvation. We praise you above any feelings we may be having. Please accept our praises to honor you, Lord Jesus, to thank you and bring glory to your name. For you are our first love Lord. We honor the place you have in our life. You are the head. You are the center of our lives. I thank you, Lord, for all the strength you give to us so we can press into the things in you.

Randy B. Brown

Written By: Thelma Conway
5 September 1983

How Great Thou Art

Oh, God, How Great Thou Art
I knew this from the start
As a child I went to Sunday School
And learned about Your Golden Rule
That if you Love Jesus and the Father, too –
A better person will be made of you

We learn by experience – so they say
But for Christ there is only ONE WAY
The way we take is up to us now
But we will get through it all somehow
With the Love and Caring from Those Above
How blessed to be enfolded in Their Love
They care so much for you and me
Aren't we lucky to have the Holy Three?

(In God is my salvation Psalm 61:7)

Practice What You Preach

On a Thursday in June 1998, the Lord reminded me what a friend once said to me, God would someday use my hands to heal people. I knew it was time to start putting into practice what God has spoken in my life. Now is the time for all of us to start acting on the prophetic words that have been spoken over us.

Today two people came to me with headaches and wanted some aspirin. I asked them if they believed God would heal the pain that is causing their headaches. One friend said "Yes!" The other one said she did not really have enough faith, but as I laid my hands on both their heads, they allowed me to pray for them. I told them God receives all the glory and honor, but it would be their faith that would allow Him to heal their headaches. It is written in scriptures *(Matthew 9:20-22)* that it is our faith that has healed us and not only our prayers. I explained that God tells us to lay hands on each other *(Mark 16:17-18)* and pray for sickness but it would be their faith that would heal them. I was so excited that God would use me to touch someone with His power in healing. Later that morning, at different times, both of my friends came to see me and tell me that their headaches went away. They did not even have to take any pills. They were both healed through their faith.

Praise God for His mighty work and His faithfulness. He receives the glory for all things! By Jesus' stripes, we are healed!

By the middle of the same afternoon, I had gotten a headache myself, and right away, I reached for my bottle of aspirin. Then the Holy Spirit reminded me *(John 14:26)* of the scriptures I had given my friends. As I sat there listening to God, I said to the Lord, "It works both ways, doesn't it, Lord?" If faith and laying hands on my friends' heads would heal their headaches, why can't I do the same thing for my own headache? It was time to put my faith into action for myself. Therefore, I laid my hands on my own head and asked the Lord to heal my headache. I decided not to take any pills but to wait on the Lord to heal me through my faith in Him. I got busy and completely forgot about my headache. It did go away and I never took any pills to help it. It took only my prayer and faith in God to relieve the pain.

I realized then that, we should always practice what we preach. When we believe for others and speak it out of our mouths, we need to hear it with our own ears what we are preaching and believe for ourselves too. What is good for one is good for all. God tells us that He is no respecter of persons *(Acts 10:34)*. He will not heal my friends and forget about me. Because God is in us, we believe that our faith will heal us. Discern the spirits *(I Corinthians 12:10)* and focus on Jesus, not our headache or illness. We should always remember to act in faith for ourselves as well as others. God is here for us just as much as He is here for others. He would not forget about one of His children. God does things in His way and in His own time. Waiting on the Lord with patience is important too. Do not give up if it does not come right away. God works in His own time.

Faith comes by hearing the word of God *(Romans 10:17)*. When you speak the word of God out of your mouth, or hear others speaking the word of God to you, learn to open up your ears and hear by faith what is being spoken. I believe the more we hear, the more faith we develop, and the more we believe. The Holy Spirit will do His part when He brings to our remembrance the word of God that is inside our heart. God is greater in us than he who is in the world *(I John*

4:4). God gives each of us a measure of faith *(Romans 12:3)* so no one is better than another in the eyes of God. The measure of faith you have or I have is the measure that God has given us. Do not compare your faith with another's. You have just the right measure for you! However, it is important to exercise that measure of faith. Faith put into action will glorify Jesus' name. Practice what you preach to others and receive it for you. Let the Lord speak to you through your own mouth when He has led you to speak to someone else. The Lord is using you to be a blessing to someone and at the same time, Jesus is blessing you. Therefore, I encourage you to start hearing your own words that you are speaking, practice what you preach, and put it into action in your own life.

Pray with me:

Father, thank you, for the measure of faith you have given me. Thank you, Lord, for your love and your mercy on my life. Lord, many times, you have spoken to me through my own mouth and I have not listened. Forgive me, Lord, and help me to practice what I speak to others. When you use me to encourage others, let me be encouraged by what you are saying to me too. Father, the words out of my mouth are spoken in faith and I want to believe for myself in faith what I believe you will do for others. You receive all the glory and honor for all my healings and I believe I am healed by my faith. Let my measure of faith grow, Lord. Let the faith I have in what I say to others be heard with my own ears. Lord, I thank you for the Holy Spirit who brings the truth to my remembrance. Thank you, Lord, for loving me and encouraging me with my own mouth. Thank you, Lord, for never leaving me and for healing my body. Thank you, Jesus, for your love and mercy.

Randy B. Brown

Written By: Thelma Conway
29 February 1996

For Jay's Dad

Remember, God hears all our prayers
And His Son, Jesus is always there.
Know that our God is testing you today
And He'll be with you all along the way!

When I go for chemo, I know it helps me live
I find strength in God, because I do believe
I always wear a smile on my face too - -
Because I'm determined, I will not be blue!

It's hard when we hurt, but God hears our plea
He will always be there for you and me.
Ask God to help you through your pain
And comfort and love you'll surely gain!

This too will pass, each day stronger you'll be
Believe me too, prayers do work, you'll see
You'll get your strength from God above
Because He'll hold you in His love!

The Night Before

(This story is dedicated to my grandchildren)

It was 24 February 1999, Wednesday; a day we call the middle of the week. The night before, three of my grandchildren, Chase Andrew, Louis James and Matthew Craig, had spent the night and we were all filled with joy in anticipation of a predicted huge snowstorm, which is very unusual for this part of North Carolina. We all looked forward to that white stuff that would cover the ground outside our homes. We were sure that the children would get out of school and we adults would not have to go to work. In our region, we do not have the proper equipment to remove snow from our streets, so everything just shuts down until the snow melts and we are able to drive on the roads again.

So much excitement filled the air. There was so much joy all around our houses. Kids ran outside just to see the flakes falling on the ground. They danced and played while their little minds were thinking, YEAH! NO SCHOOL TOMORROW! We working adults were also thinking as the little children were, YEAH! NO WORK TOMORROW!

The next morning when we expected to see all that snow, somehow the clouds that would bring the snow did not form. No phone calls were made to employees, even though the TV spoke of potential school and workplace closings, as the first snowflakes began to fall. As I lay in my bed, I waited for the phone to ring, still expecting my boss to say, "NO WORK TODAY!" Nevertheless, as time went on, it was getting late and I knew I had to get up. I went on to work, still hearing that there was a chance of snow in our area. Soon they were telling us we might only get one inch of snow. BIG DEAL, I thought. The night before was so much more fun; with the delight of thinking there would be a day off in the middle of the week! Thank God for the joy of anything that He gives us. Whether or not we get our own way, the joy of the Lord still fills our heart each day with Him.

Even though we all had to carry on with normal routines of work and school, joy still came because God showed me how blessed we really are. Our very jobs are a blessing from Him! When you do not feel like laughing, let God help you laugh with His joy. Look around you right now and see all that is happening in your life with the things you have. Your homes, your cars, your children, spouses, your jobs, maybe even a simple thing as a park bench someone can rest on. God always gives us so much that we need to be thankful for *(I Chronicles 16:34, Psalm 100:4-5, I Thessalonians 5:16-18 and Colossians 3:15)*. The Bible tells us to be thankful for all things, even the little things. So even though the night before we were all excited and thanking God for an anticipated snowfall which did not come, we still understand that our joy is not in material things, but in God's spiritual gifts. Our joy comes from the Lord. Joy is in everything because everything comes from God in the first place.

What we need to do is be filled with the things God gives us in everyday life, for example, our jobs. Many people are unemployed. We need to start looking up and be thankful that we have a job. We have joy when we see someone we do not even know smiling at us. That comes from the Lord. He is always sending someone to cheer up our down times. Look at someone and give him or her one of your smiles to brighten up their day. You never know when God will send someone to you for a little bit of His love. Share the Lord with someone today and see the joy of the Lord fill the atmosphere around you with His presence. That is the real joy, being in the presence of God as He fills the air around you. There is joy and peace just being in His presence. The joy of the Lord is our strength *(Nehemiah 8:10, John 15:10)* and we are to be filled with the joy of the Lord. We do not always recognize God's joy because we are too busy watching earthly things to give us happiness.

Let us pray:

Thank you, Father, for the blood that gives me salvation and frees me from sin. Thank you for dying for me. Jesus, I am because you are. Father, to you I give thanks for all the things you have given to me and are still going to give to me. I thank you for my job. Lord, for those that do not work I thank you that they can be at home. I thank you for my home, for my family, and for my friends. Lord, I thank you for the jobs you are creating right now for the ones who need them. I pray that you would fill me with your joy and peace and reveal to my spirit the things that bring you joy. I want to laugh with you, Jesus. I want to be filled with the presence of God and His holy joy. I thank you, Father, even for the things I do not have. I know that everything comes from you and I have all that I need in you, Lord. Thank you, Lord. I pray in Jesus' name. I thank you, Lord.

Randy B. Brown

Written By: Thelma M. B. Conway
5 May 1953

What is Life?

Tell me what is the meaning of life,
Is it full of sorrow, or full of strife?
With everyone aiming for just one thing - -
To end up where God's Angels sing?

What is life, if you feel blue,
Struggling along, just for you?
Can't you see, there's more than one –
There's lots of work that's left undone!

What is life, if you live only for you
Your life is empty, lonely and blue!
So, let's cheer up, there's a future ahead
Be glad you're alive, instead of dead.

There is more than you in this world, you know
You have to learn to reap what you sow.
Hold up your head, look up to God above,
Surely, you'll see what is meant by His love!

What is life if you turn things away?
You may feel good, but you have to pay!
Start now to live, start now to show - -
You can hold your head high wherever you go!

Life is what you make it, so they say
You live for tomorrows, not for today!
Forget yesteryears, forever look ahead
Don't look back, you'll be sorry you did.

What is life, if you're always blue and sad?
You just make yourself and others feel bad.
Are you helping yourself by doing this?
Getting sorrow, instead of joy and bliss?

Hold your head high, life is worth living - -
Try to be you, and try to start giving.
You'll be glad that you did; so try today
Hold your head high, and be proud to say:

WHAT IS LIFE? WHY, LIFE IS THE BEST!
Always striving to take the test –
I'm glad I'm alive, can you truthfully say:
GEE, "BUT I'M GLAD TO BE LIVING TODAY!"

The Sweetness of the Scriptures

It was early in the morning on 14 May, my oldest daughter's birthday. As I was typing, I glanced at the file cabinet in my office and noticed the box of Sweet Tart candies sitting on top of it. The Holy Spirit took me into my secret place with the Lord, while He showed me God's heart for His Word, the BIBLE.

The candy in this box is wrapped in individual pieces and the wrappers have a scripture on them. Whenever anyone comes in looking for candy, I have only one rule: they must read the scripture before they eat the candy. That way, they will be blessed by what God has to say to them today. Those who have taken a piece of that candy have all read the scriptures, and sometimes I receive a comment, but at least they read God's Word. Not one person in the building has ever taken a piece without standing there and reading the scripture in front of me. I get blessed just watching God bless them. However, not all will receive what God has to say to them. They read because they want the candy, but do not understand the blessing it is wrapped in. I just pray that it would seep into their spirits, and they would feel the love God wants to give to them at that particular moment in their life.

This is what the Lord revealed to me about that box of candy. God spoke and I listened. As He revealed to me through His Holy Spirit, I heard Him say that many will read His scriptures and receive His love, but there are always some who read the scripture just because someone asked them to. They will not receive anything but that candy melting in their mouth. They will taste of the sweetness of candy, but not the sweetness in God's scriptures. The Lord showed me in that candy box the sweetness of His Word. He inspired the scriptures so we would know Him as a Father, a lover, and a friend and as our King. Many do not understand what a friend is, or what the role of a father is. A father is someone who teaches you the way to do things right, and what you are doing wrong. A father gives direction and guidance for living, making sure nothing but the best is given for his children. Many do not understand what a king is. A king is a ruler who makes all the rules for his kingdom to live by. If you do not live by his rules, you lose and are locked out of the kingdom forever. A friend is someone who loves you and cares what is happening to you. A friend will watch out for your best interest, making sure he or she is available at all times to be there if you need someone to talk to. A lover is someone you want to be with all the time. You go out of your way to please him or her by giving gifts, quality time, and words of encouragement. A lover is someone you trust with your deepest dark secrets. A lover is someone you know loves you unconditionally no matter what you do, who stands by you and cares for you. If you love someone you may not like what he or she is doing, but you are there loving that person through all his or her mistakes. You never give up on them, because you love them. God says He is all these things, wrapped into one spirit that dwells within our soul. God is our everything. All you need to do is read His Word to know Him. God showed me that many just do not read His Word. They may pick up the Bible because someone is watching them, or they have it lying around on one of their tables in the home, possibly even in their office, as a "decoration". God wants us to use His Word, not as a decoration or symbol, but for guidance, direction, and wisdom and to know His love for His children. He wants to show you His Kingdom, His love for you, and the way to eternal life with His Son. God's love is so much sweeter than that candy on my cabinet or any table. When I look at that box of candy I don't just see the box of candy, I see the scripture too. That candy is wrapped in words that are life to my spirit; they are God's words for living; they encourage me and lift up my spirit. Yes, God's Word is sweet and it is life to all our spirits. If we do not pick it up and read it, we will never know whom God is and what Jesus did for us. We will never have the Holy Spirit to fill us with His presence and teach us His ways. If we do not tell others about the sweetness in God's Word, they may never know how much He loves them and what a friend He can be to them.

Pick up your Bible and read it, for it is your lifesaver, a way to God Himself, His Kingdom, and your eternal home through Jesus His only Son, our Lord, Master, and most of all our Savior. Jesus died for all our sins, no matter what we did. We are forgiven through the Blood of Christ *(John 3:16-17),* and there is no other way to God except through the Blood of Christ *(John 14:6)*. So, you see, Jesus is the only way, the truth, and the life. God did not write the scriptures for only a few. He wrote them for everyone. God showed me that many just throw away the paper off that candy and do not even take in what they just read, because they just do not know Him *(John 14:7)* and what He wants to tell them. Everyday, God has something to say, every moment He is waiting to talk with us.

Do not let another day go by without picking up your Bible from the table and letting the Holy Spirit show you what Jesus did for you. Pick it up and let God talk to you. It is a mystery, a love letter, and a book of guidance and direction for life. The Bible is God's candy box; it is sweetness to your spirit. Eat His candy and live with purpose and direction. Come to the Cross and invite Jesus into your heart, be filled with the Holy Spirit and start your new journey with the sweetness of God's gift to you in His Word. Watch your life go from glory to glory because you have finally tasted God's Word. God is waiting for His children to start reading and receiving. Come, read and receive, no longer stand for just knowing what the Bible says, receive what Jesus has done for you. Jesus is waiting for you. Won't you come and know my Jesus? Won't you receive what God says you are to Him? Let God show you what He thinks. Man only has opinions, but God is truth and He never lies *(Hebrews 6:17-18)*. He cannot lie. He keeps all His promises, as we are told in the scriptures, but you will not know unless you pick up your Bible and read the sweetness of His Scriptures. He is waiting! Come and receive ALL that He has for you. I pray that you will know my Jesus as your lover and friend. He is the best friend you will ever have! God bless you and have a wonderful journey into God's Word! Eat of the sweetness of His Scriptures. Let His word melt in your heart and build your lifeline into God's love, mercy, and grace.

Let me pray with you now:

Oh Lord, Father in Heaven, our Holy Heavenly Father, creator of creation and of all things, I come to you right now and ask you to forgive me of all my sins. Cleanse me by the Blood of Christ and open up my heart that I will receive all that you have for me in your Word. I need your guidance and direction in my life. I want to be a vessel to honor Jesus who saved me and gave me eternal life. Lord, I know I have done a lot of wrong things and made many wrong choices in my life, even thoughts that flow through my mind are not what I truly want in my head, but I know that you are a God of miracles and a God who loves and forgives me, so I am reaching to you now. I ask you to let the sweetness of your scriptures change my life. Help me to love others as you have commanded me to do. I ask you to flow inside my body and guide me, show me which way you would have me to go. Lord, I thank you for saving me. I thank you for forgiving me. I thank you for the mercy and grace you always give me. I pray that I will forgive others and give mercy and grace to them. I need your hand in my life leading me, so I ask you to have your way with me, in Jesus' name. I ask you right now to lead, guide, and direct my path and help me to completely trust in you for all things, in Jesus' name. Thank you Lord.

Randy B. Brown

Written By: Thelma Conway
13 June 1996

How Strong is my Faith?

My Dearest Lord, in Your Heaven, up above
Please look down on my Daughter with abundance of Love.

She struggles today with Knowing You
And I tell her she does have Faith, too.

Help her in her daily walk each day
That You won't let anything get in her way.

She loves You so much, Lord, she does You know
And always to people, it really does show!

Learning about the Holy Spirit is what she does now
In her walk, Lord Jesus, keep on helping her somehow.

"Jesus Sees the Value in Every Person" – my Pastor said today
You know that is a "Powerful Saying" he sent our way!

Remember, for encouragement you don't have to look far
Look up towards the Heavens, and talk to a star.

Also, let Jesus be your guide – He is Your Friend
He will take you to His Heart – again and again!

Lord, take care of my child, hug her tight,

And always, please keep her in Your Sight!

The Fountain of Life

It was a cool morning in May of 2001, and I sat waiting to hear from God while my two dogs kept coming in the room wanting my attention. I began to get upset because I was trying to focus on God and what He wanted to show me. Here I am waiting to hear from the Lord and these jealous dogs keep interrupting my thoughts! As I put my focus back on the Lord, He began to speak into my spirit.

I watched these dogs come in for my attention and I saw the jealousy in both of them, each one wanting to be the first to get my attention. The Lord showed me how sometimes we, His creation, act just like my dogs were. We fight for His attention too! Sure, we all want His attention, and when we see Him doing something in someone else we may get jealous. We leave His presence, and then we go back and forth into His presence again, hoping He will respond. The dogs finally stood in front of me, waiting for me to say or do something to show them I was recognizing their presence, wondering whom I would respond to first. A pat on the head or even a kiss on the head would have made them happy. We, too, wait for God's attention, for a kiss, a pat in our heart, and even for His presence. We wait just for Him to notice we are there, waiting to see if He loves us or if He will speak. We leave His presence many times because we do not wait long enough for Him to respond. We leave discouraged and go back and forth until we get a response. If we will wait on God to answer, He will, but in His time. Be still and know that He is God *(Psalm 46:10)*. We do not have to fight for His attention; He loves everyone unconditionally.

My eyes were led to a dying plant on my porch. It looked as if it had a little life in it still, but was waiting for me to feed it water. It was dry and needed much water to live. It had many bad leaves hanging off it, although there was still life inside it. There were a few fresh new leaves. Without water and proper attention, it would eventually die. However, the plant was struggling to hold on to life on its own. If we are not doing anything with our relationship with you, Lord, we die from lack of spiritual water. We too struggle to hang on to life on our own. Now I know the plant cannot cry out for help, but we certainly can. If we will just open our mouths and yell JESUS! I know He will be there. However, like the dogs, we wait and leave and then come back again and wait, only to be disappointed because we did not wait long enough in His presence to feel Him or hear His voice. When we wait, we will be satisfied. If we set aside a special time just to be with His Word and be in His presence, we will walk away with a fresh new hope in our spirits. However, there are times we may have come only long enough for a pat on the head and we do not wait for the kiss from His lips or His arms wrapped around us. Sometimes we are too busy with other things. The water our souls need does not come, and we go away only to struggle for life, hanging on to our own understanding instead of reaching and waiting for God and His understanding. When we give the plant water, it lives. When we allow God's Word to feed us, we live. Do not walk away empty hearted because you did not wait in God's presence long enough for Him to answer you.

Our houses, our temples that belong to God are safe. They are sealed by the Holy Spirit *(Ephesians 1:13-14 and Ephesians 4:30)* and washed in the Blood of the Lamb and nothing can take us from the hand of God, not even man *(John 10:27-30)*. We are covered by the glory rain of God and fed by the life in His breath. We breathe only because of the Cross. We have life only because of the Cross.

Praise God, and thank you, Jesus for the Cross.

God's fountain of life is reading His Word each day and sitting in His presence waiting to hear His voice revealing Himself to us. Drink from His fountain of life and live to serve Him, for He is a Holy God and a worthy Lord. This life we live is His creation, not ours. We exist because He is. Do not look at others to see what God is doing in them. Start looking to see what God is doing in you. He does things differently with each person. We are all His children, unique to Him. We are all different parts of the body of Christ, designed to do different things. God created each of us for His purpose to be used for His plan *(Romans 8:28)*. You must be placed where God places you. Be what He created you to be. Do what He put in your spirit to do. Look to God's fountain of Life for your spiritual watering, let His Holy goodness love, feed, and fill you so you can live for His glory. God, He is our Fountain of Life.

Let me pray with you now:

Lord, it is time we wait in your presence. I pray you put a desire in all our spirits not to be rushed but to linger in your presence. Lord, we are waiting and longing for a kiss, not just a pat on the head from your hand, but life from your drinking fountain. I pray we drink from your fountain of life so we can live with energy to serve our Holy God. We will not have to struggle if we just give you time to answer, so we are waiting for your answer, Lord. Father, feed, water, pat, kiss us, all your children. Fill us with living water from your fountain of life, in Jesus' name. Bring the glory rain and the golden sunshine to our spirits, your spirit living in us. Let us walk in the life of your word and not in the death of the world. Father, draw us all to your fountain of life, in Jesus' name. Help us, Lord, to stand at the foot of the Cross and wait to hear your voice. Then we will drink and you can fill us with your Holy Spirit, in Jesus' name. Lord, put a thirst in our spirits to reach for you and to wait until we hear from your lips. Thank you, Lord, for always being there for us. I love the way you talk to us in your own unique ways. I heard you, Lord, and I drank from your Holy Fountain of Life today. You have filled me with your spiritual water once again. Then I can live and not struggle to hang on, but truly be energized in your word. You are wonderful, LORD! Thank you, Jesus. Oh Father, shower us with your glory rain. Fill us with all of you, in Jesus' name. Thank you, Lord, for we have new life in our bones because of the spiritual fountain of God!

Written By: Thelma Conway
3 April 1973

Boy Lost

You strayed away from the ties that bound you
Thinking that the people who now surround you
Are much better than the ones you left behind - -
Please open your eyes wide – Son, you cannot be so blind.

The folks at home – their heart break more every day
Wondering what went wrong, as each night they silently pray

Lord above, please let Your love protect him along life's way
Help him to see and understand – we wanted him so to stay!
May he know, though far away – he may think he's content
He turned our world upside-down, the day he so calmly went!

Watching Over His Creation

It was the month of June 2001 and a beautiful morning in the Lord. As I was sitting on the porch with two of my grandchildren, watching them play with the blocks and waiting for their mom to pick them up for school, I saw a little blue jay come to one of many birdhouses we had fastened on our fence. The blue jay poked his head in as if to check things out and make sure his house was safe. Than he went and sat on the side of the fence by that house, so he could keep watch over it and what was inside. As I reflected on what God wanted to tell me, I felt in my spirit the Lord was showing me about our houses, our temples of Him, our bodies. As the blue jay watches over his house to see that it is untouched and nothing gets in it except what he has put there, we too should watch over our house (our spirits) so they remain untouched by the world. We should put only the things of God in His temple. Get rid of the things we put in the temple that are in the world. We are to guard our bodies with His Holy Spirit and protect them from things coming in that are not of Christ. We must guard ourselves against the temptations of the flesh *(Matthew 26:41)*. We are to be focused on Jesus; come to His house, read His Word, and be filled with fresh thoughts. When thoughts come that are not of God we must ask ourselves, before we do anything, "What would Jesus do if He were here with me now?" and act accordingly by His Spirit. Wake up the Spirit of God within us, for His Word says He is greater who is in us *(I John 4:4)*.

The Lord showed me that if we look at the negative, we cannot see Him in truth. God touches us in many ways to let us know He is near. We do not always see that because we let the lies of the devil feed our thoughts. When we know God's Word, we know truth, and we must rebuke the lies, in Jesus' name. Jesus gave us authority to do that and we must take that authority with boldness and belief. It is in faith that the mountains will move *(Matthew 17:20)* and in faith we grow closer to God. Our body houses the spirit of God. He gave us life and breathed into our nostrils the air we live on. We cannot see the air and yet we are breathing it. We believe it will be there for us to use so we can live. Actually, I do not even think we worry about it not being there. We have faith in something we do not even see. Jesus died for us in human form, but because we were not there, some of us struggle believing He ever existed. We believe the lies of the enemy telling us that we cannot see Him. Yet we believe in history books. We were not there, but we believe in man's account of the past.

God's book, the Bible, is His love letter to us and we believe in it by faith. Without faith *(Matthew 21:21-22)* we have nothing because faith is hope, hope is the unseen that we believe in without seeing. We have no hope for the future without faith. It is in faith that we allow His spirit to flow through us and if we will focus on His spirit in us, we will remember who we belong to, Jesus, not the world.

Just like the little blue jay stood watch over his house, I believe God stands watch over all His houses, yet we do not always know He is there. To feel safe in Him we must remember God is always there watching over us whether we feel Him or not, whether we see Him or not. Believe in His Word, His truth, His history book, and His love letter to us. He is there! He says He will never leave us *(Hebrews 13:5)*.

You see, there are so many things God wants to tell us if we will just listen. He will tell us everything He wants us to know. We have to listen first to hear, than believe in faith that it is God speaking to us.

I started listening to Him, and I can tell you it is the most loving experience of faith. Our human minds can not imagine this wonderful journey were on. I believe it and know it is He as He deposits it in my spirit, His spirit that dwells within my body. I must always remember to thank Him. I must respect the things He shows me and believe it is He doing it. God would never lie; He is the Father of Truth, Hope, and Peace. Because of Jesus and His death on the Cross, we have hope and should know it is the truth; yet peace does not always come because of the lies in our thoughts. Rebuke those lies of Satan, who is the father of lies *(John 8:44)*, and focus on God who is truth *(John 1:14 and John 17:17)*. In that, focus the peace will come, and then the joy will fill your soul, because joy comes when peace is present. If we rest our thoughts on God, He will give us discernment by His Holy Spirit and He will show us many things. He spoke to me one day eating popcorn. Listen to your heart. Is it God, or is it Satan, you want to believe? There is no comparison. Our spirits will know, because we are born again and we belong to Jesus now, not the world *(Galatians 2:20)*.

Life gives you many pleasures from the world and they are only temporary. Only God can give you heavenly pleasure and promises that are permanent. So we must decide. Is it the world and temporary things we want, or is it eternity and a permanent home in glory that we want? Praise God, for He has given us a second chance at life through the Blood of Christ. We can be born again and make the right choices and have eternal life with HIM! It is all in your faith! Have FAITH in Christ and BELIEVE it is GOD!

I want God alone, watching over my house and me. I put my faith and trust in Him. He is an all-knowing God and He loves us. You cannot hide from Him as the little blue jay hid from his children, for God sees everything. He sits next to us and watches over His temple and the things inside it. You will feel His presence when you look

His way. He is always there watching us.

Please let me pray with you:

Lord, oh most holy heavenly Father, thank you for watching over us and being there even when we do not feel you. Lord, you are always with us, for your word tells us you never leave us. Father, I lift up everyone reading this story, and pray that you will continue to keep watch over every step they take in Jesus' name. Build our faith and make us stronger, Father, give us revelations of you in everything we look at that comes from heaven. As we see things that are of you, I pray that we will hear your voice speak things to our spirits what you would have us know. Father, let our eyes continually focus on you and your word in Jesus' name. I pray, Lord, that we would feel your presence and know you are right beside us keeping watch over us in all that we do, in Jesus' name. Father, it is in your truth we believe. We pray for discernment to rebuke the lies of the enemy. Build our spirits, Lord, with your word and your grace. Thank you, Father, for the truth in your word. Thank you, Father, for the Holy Spirit who leads us into all truth. Thank you, Lord, for you, oh God, are holy and powerful and mighty. It is in Jesus' name we pray.

Written By: Thelma Conway
26 March 1983

Peace

"I HAVE PEACE IN MY HEART" today
"BECAUSE HE LIVES," again I say
Remember, "ALONG THE ROAD" – I know Thee
"EACH STEP OF THE WAY," Jesus says" "FOLLOW ME."

"HE LOOKED BEYOND MY FAULT" and made me whole
He is the "HEALER OF BROKEN HEART" – so I am told
"HOW LONG HAS IT BEEN?" since you prayed to Him
and let Him wash you clean from sin?

You know "JESUS IS COMING SOON," we know this to be true
"SOMETHING BEAUTIFUL" will happen then to me and you
So, "WHEN WE SEE CHRIST" – what a glorious day it will be
So "FILL MY CUP LORD," because "I WILL SERVE THEE!"

"HE'LL UNDERSTAND AND SAY 'Well Done'" – to me

Because "I'M HIS, HE'S MINE" don't you see?
I want to "REACH OUT AND TOUCH HIM" along the way
So "BLESSED REDEEMER," please help me today.

"THANK YOU, GOD, FOR THE PROMISE OF SPRING"
And all the warmth of love it will bring
"I'LL TELL THE WORLD" to let us all shout and sing
So the bells in the "MANSION OVER THE HILLTOP" will ring!

Keep Your Focus on Me

(This story is dedicated to Kathy Peterpaul)

One morning in October 2001, it was a glorious day in the Lord. As I got up and dressed for work, I was not able to put on my pearl and gold chain necklace, so I grabbed it and carried it in my hand out to the car. I figured that someone at work would be able to help me with it. When I arrived at work and got out of the car, I realized I had left the necklace in the vehicle, so I went back to get it. I walked into the office, put my things down on my desk, and went in to see my boss. When I got back to my desk, I remembered it was what we call POTATO DAY! I ran around checking with everyone to see who wanted potatoes, and never noticed I did not have my necklace on yet. After the major task was done, I was able to focus on getting my things put away. It was then I realized my necklace was missing.

The search was on. My boss and many other co-workers started retracing my footsteps trying to find the lost necklace. We emptied out my purse and travel bag and there was no necklace. Many were telling me that I was crazy, that I left it at home and never had it with me in the first place. They said when I get home I would be very surprised when I see it there. They joked about calling the doctors to tell them I needed help. I started to wonder. Was I wrong, did I or did I not bring it in? I was certain I had, but I got confused and started to believe them. This was becoming a good lesson in God's Word: do not be deceived by false prophets! I listened to others, got confused, and started believing them instead of trusting what I knew was the truth *(Luke 21:8)*.

I went to our copy room to search again. By this time, I figured it would show up at home, and the office staff must be right about leaving it at home. The Holy Spirit urged me to seek God. While on my knees looking under the copy machine and the table I looked up and said, "Lord, I know that it is just a material thing and that you can take anything you want because it belongs to you in the first place. I also know that you, Jesus, can see that necklace and know right where it is, so please show me." I got up, went into the hallway, and headed back to my desk knowing that Jesus would open my eyes to find that necklace soon. All of a sudden coming down the hall was my friend Kathy. I could not see her face and body, because all I saw was my necklace hanging around her neck. That necklace was so bright and stood out like something I never had seen before, it was so beautiful. The pearls were so white and bright and the gold links in between each pearl was so bright! I walked up to her and said, "Is that my necklace you have on?" Kathy said, "Yes, I was wondering when you would start looking for it and I even forgot it was around my neck!" She had seen it on my desk and took it for a joke, because I had left it there unattended.

I went back to my desk and held the necklace under my fingers and looked up at God and said, "Thank you, Lord, I knew you would find it, just thank you, thank you Lord!" After I settled in and started working I heard the Holy Spirit speaking to me. In my spirit, He revealed the meaning behind the things that took place this morning. God showed me that my focus lately had not been on Him first but on things around me. I had already gone in to see Kathy once this morning to say hi, and I never saw that necklace on her. She even made it a point to let me see the necklace around her neck, but I never once noticed it because I was too involved in my own thoughts.

I believe that God was saying, when we focus on Him, He has

many things to show us and tell us. He is always there, but we do not always notice Him because we are so busy with the things around us. We are busy focusing on what we are walking through and what we want from the world. Our focus becomes confused and we miss Him in many things He shows us. We know who God is and that He is always there, but I believe often we take Him for granted and only cry out to Him when we cannot figure things out for ourselves. Why can't we just stop and seek Him first, as He directs us in His Word? He will show us all things that we have a need for *(Matthew 6:33, Matthew 7:7)*. When our focus is on the Lord, I believe our days run smoother and we are far less frustrated. We need to focus on God first. Then, the things around us will easily fall into place. We are to be led by the Holy Spirit who guides us to the things of God.

I know that necklace was valuable in a worldly sense, but in the eyes of God, it was not as valuable as what He wanted me to do that morning. Here I was running around seeking that expensive necklace, when God Himself is much more valuable than any gold or pearl in the world. All I had to do was stop and get my focus back on the things above that are eternal and priceless, and Jesus would have taken care of the necklace. When we lose something in the world that is precious to us, we forget that the giver is more precious than the gift. We must learn to help each other and encourage each other to seek first the Kingdom of God. Then all things will be added unto us *(Matthew 6:33)*. Jesus left His Spirit behind to help us during times we need comfort or help. The Holy Spirit is our comforter and our guide in this present world. He will help us keep our focus on the things above when we seek the Lord first and ask Him to come. We must invite the Holy Spirit to come, for He is a gentleman and will not push Himself on us. Let us give Him free reign to come first thing each morning before we have to experience any frustrations.

God is good and He wants every good thing for us. I learned a big lesson about keeping my eyes on the Lord and off what I can do on my own. If I had put God first, I might have seen that necklace earlier, and not everyone would have been inconvenienced looking for it with me. When I first noticed it missing, I should have stopped right then and asked God to forgive me for putting potatoes before Him. When I went into Kathy's room, the first time God would have shown me that necklace and all that running around would not have been necessary. Now even though it was a joke for Kathy to take the necklace off my desk, I am grateful she did, because I learned a good lesson. Nothing is more important or more precious than my relationship with Jesus.

There will be many times when we are walking through things when our focus will be elsewhere, but if we can learn to stop before going too far, look up, and seek God first, He will send the Holy Spirit to help us through everything we face. "Keep your focus on Me", is what the Lord spoke to me about this day. When I did stop and look up it only took about three seconds before He opened my eyes to the truth in that whole situation. First, I was not confused about leaving that necklace at home. I was right; I did bring it into work. Originally, I even forgot I left it in the car and went back to get it out. However, the devil can easily deceive us with confusion if our focus is not on God first. Therefore, confusion was taken away and the truth was revealed when my focus was right. I was not focused on God first, but when I did, He was there taking care of the things around me and the truth was revealed to us all. I encourage you to practice focusing on God first in everything and help those around you to do the same thing. God tells us to encourage each other in our faith *(Romans 8:12)*. Keep your focus on Him!

Let us pray:

Father, I thank you that you are faithful and you have given us the Lord Jesus to save us. Even when you took Him home with you, Lord, you did not leave us comfortless; you left us the Holy Spirit. Thank you, Lord, that we can encourage each other in our faith and that you are always present to help us whenever we ask for your help. Father, I pray that I would focus first on you and that the Holy Spirit would lead me each day with the things you lay out before me. I thank you, Lord that you go before me and prepare the way before I even take a step in that direction. Father, I pray that my focus would be on the things eternal and not earthly. Lord, I believe you will show me all the things I need to know as long as I seek first your Kingdom. Forgive me, Lord, for the times I have missed you because my focus was not on you first. I thank you that you always bring me back in right standing with you. Help me to be still and know that you are my God. Help me to be an encourager to those around me, and help us to focus first on You, Lord. In Jesus' name, I pray and give thanks.

Written By: Thelma Conway
25 February 1968

Courage

The days go swiftly by, my Son, though you are far away
But be it known you are in my thoughts every single day
And when I, at times, may feel lonely or seem a little blue
I read over your cards and letters and feel so close to you.

This month has almost gone, Son, never again to return
Many things life has taught me, as each day I learn
More to accept life for what it is – trying not to look back
We must believe things can't for long be dreary and black.

Time changes many things, though some things we cannot change
ever
God gives us courage to stand our pains, helps us go ahead forever.
We must accept life as it is, and try not to keep looking back
Though at times we feel that even courage – we really do lack.

If God loves us, so shall we trust and believe in Him always
And hope and pray for everyone for there will be brighter days.
We have our dreams, our hopes, the future should be bright
And many is the time we wonder – how we got through last night!

They say, "time heals all wounds" – I wonder, does it really, my
Son?
Oh, yes, if we believe in God above, we will know again that we
have won.
Our heartaches are just Gods' test – to prove if we are weak or

strong

And ahead we must always surge – for we cannot stay weak for
long!

Yes, life at times is very hard, the pains that we must bear
But better people we will be, if we all do our fair share
So, here's to you, my Sailor, may God protect you with His Love
And may the Angels, always, shine on you from Heaven, above!

God, please keep my Sailor safe and protect him every day
Keep him healthy, happy, and strong while he is so far away
Thank you, God, for everything – no matter how large or small
We all give Thanks to Thee, for You will never let us fall!

Look at the Light
Through the Darkness

(This story is dedicated to Jackie Hornage)

It was such a dark and cloudy day on Thursday, 29 August 2002. It had been raining off and on all week long. I had been taking a supervisory skills training class all week at work and today, the last day of class, the facilitators worked hard to finish up so we could leave early. As I was driving home, I watched some very dark clouds, hoping I would get home before the pouring rain came. The Lord started talking to me about His light being all around me, even in the darkness of these clouds. God was telling me to look through the darkness in the clouds and see His light around me because He never leaves me nor forsakes me *(Hebrews 13:5)*. This is what God wanted me to be looking at and thinking about, but I had other things on my mind. I was thinking how I needed to hurry home before the rain poured down and I could not see to drive. No! God wanted to show me something about Him first. He wanted me to hear His voice. The Holy Spirit began teaching me to trust and have faith in who God is, instead of looking at my situation and fearing the storm that is about to come. The Holy Spirit kept directing my attention to look up at the whole sky all around me. The sky was very dark. There was one black cloud in the shape of a bat. Its wings were spread out as if it were flying around watching the earth. God was talking to me about seeing His light through the darkness in my own life. I was listening and looking with such awe at all, He was showing me. I got so excited I called Jackie, our secretary at church at the time of this writing. She has always read the stories God has given me and she has been so encouraged by them. This time I wanted to share a story with her as it was happening so I called her and ask if I could come see her. She was busy, but told me to please come; she would love to see me.

While driving to the church the Lord was speaking so much to me that I got concerned that I would not be able to remember all He was showing me before I could share it with Jackie. I asked God to please, wait until I get to Jackie. I wanted her to see the story with her own eyes this time and share in His glory. God is so gracious. I got to the church and asked Jackie to come outside. I felt led to share this story with her as God was speaking it to me.

I asked Jackie to look up and tell me what she saw. Jackie said, "A dark sky." I said, "Jackie, look closer at that sky and all around us and tell me, what do you really see when you look at those dark clouds in the sky that surround us?" She said, "I don't know, except that it looks like it is going to pour down rain any minute."

God began speaking much louder and so clearly, I could hear His voice. I begin to share with Jackie what I saw and what I believed God was saying. I said, "Jackie, you always read my stories and have encouraged me with your excitement of the revelations they bring. God is going to let you see this story happen right before your very own eyes. The Holy Spirit directed me to show you what God is revealing to me as I looked at that dark ugly sky. So here goes! I want you to look at the sky while I tell you." Jackie was smiling and excited as she waited to see what God had to say. That encouraged me even more just watching her excitement and anticipation.

As Jackie and I were looking up at the sky and the clouds, some of them were very dark clouds, some of the clouds were black, and some were varied shades of gray. I believed God wanted us to see something through His eyes, not our own, as we looked at that sky.

The Lord wants us to be at peace and rest in all our situations we go through. God tells us not to worry but to trust in Him *(Matthew 6:25-28a)*. I felt in my spirit God wanted to share the beauty of what He sees in all this darkness surrounding us. God wanted us to see His light through all that darkness.

The sky was very dark in some places but you could see these rays of light in some of the clouds. Even though the sky was dark, we could still see light through the holes that were in some of the cloud formations. Looking straight ahead of us with the storm coming, we could see God's light through the darkness as it was shining down in rays on the earth. As we looked ahead right in front of our eyes, there was a beautiful crystal blue sky. The sun was peeping through and made it look so bright. The sky had fluffy white clouds all through it so you knew that there was light and victory at the end of the storm surrounding us. God revealed to me what I believe He wanted us to see. When you are in a storm, it may seem light at times, seem dark at other times, and look as if the darkness will never end, but if we keep our eyes focused on Him, He has already taken care of the situation. The victory has already been won so we should not worry about what we think we see now. Jesus said it was finished when he died on the Cross for our sins *(John 19:30)*. All we have to do is believe, trust, and keep our eyes focused on the Lord. Then the Lord said to me, "While you're walking through your storms, focus on Me and not the situations you're walking in. The darkness may look bad and even may look as if it is getting ready to pour all over you, but you can see more and more light as you keep walking toward My light that is ahead of you." God was saying we should keep running the race and finish the battle *(Hebrews 12:1)*. The battle is already won; Jesus took care of it years ago on the Cross. We just have to walk through the storm. As we do, we will grow closer to Him.

Our faith will be built on solid ground. God said to me, "Satan cannot be everywhere, but I am all around you at all times, I will never leave you nor forsake you *(Hebrews 13:5)*. I do not lie and I never change *(Malachi 3:6)*, I am with you always. Satan has to send his demons to watch the world because he cannot be everywhere. They watch, see what is going on, then they run back to him, giving him their report. However, while Satan is telling his demons what to do next, you may already be through your battle because your eyes were focused on Me, your Heavenly Father. The demons did not have enough time to run, give their report to Satan, and get their next assignment before you have walked through the storm. You have kept your focus and won the race that was set before you *(Hebrews 12:1)*. The toughest and darkest part of the battle was over because in My Word, I tell you to obey my commandments, resist the devil and he will flee from you *(James 4:6-7)*. Randy, Jackie, because your eyes are focused on Me, not the world and your situation, you can see my light through all the darkness. You win because My Son finished the battle before you were even born." Wow, that was a powerful revelation to me!

"Telling this story needs a picture," Jackie said. This is one of those beautiful revelations God gives, and that makes your mind overwhelmed. It is amazing to see it and hear Him speak, while looking at His lesson unfolding right before your eyes. It is so wonderful you cannot describe the experience of being in His presence, hearing His voice, and watching it take place, all at the same time. We did not want to leave. It was so awesome looking at that dark sky, knowing the big storm was about to come, but we could see the light and the victory ahead and knew we had won the battle by looking to the light of God Himself.

I have been walking through a very heavy storm for the last year, and my focus was on my situation and not my Creator. God was talking to me through it all, but I had not been listening or receiving His blessings. I was hearing but I was not listening. While Jackie and I were finishing our conversation, a butterfly flew right between our faces. It was so close to our faces that we had to take a step backwards to get out of the way. We knew God was telling us something and confirming what we just experienced. I believe many Christians are hearing God but not listening to Him and they are stuck in a cocoon. God wants to bring them out and show His beauty. That must be what the butterfly symbolized as it flew between us. This beautiful butterfly is coming out of her cocoon! I pray you too will come out of the cocoon you find yourself in, and not only will you hear God speaking to you, but that you will listen and act on what He is showing you. God has always been there, all around us in the mist of our storms. Many times we have been clouded by the world and the situations we are in, not keeping our eyes focused on Him, His Word, all the teachings we have had, and the prophecies that have been spoken over us.

At the time of the storm, I could not see the whole picture of God's glory. I could not see God's greatness. I could not even see who He is in me and who I am in Him. The world and the things I was walking through had clouded my thinking. What an awesome Holy God we have that He never, ever gives up on us. Trust and faith in God must be put into action in our lives and our situations. When we take our eyes off our problems, the storm surrounding us with its dark clouds, and focus instead on who Jesus is in us, I know we can see His light through the darkness.

I have learned through this experience that our relationship with God is the most precious thing we will ever own. We must be careful to protect it and keep our focus on God alone. As you go through the storm, thank Him for what He did on the Cross just for you. Let

God put life back in your spirit. Allow the Holy Spirit to be your friend and walk you through the tough times. He knows the end of the battle. God gave us his Spirit to be our helper and comforter, to guide us into peace in the midst of the storm. Satan does not know the end because he is hoping we will not see God through the storm. He will work very hard to stop us from making it to the finish line *(Luke 22:29-32)*. So keep your focus and see what God will do, in and through you, as you trust Him. Have faith to believe He is with you all the way and all the time. Trust the spirit in you that is greater than all your problems and trials. Walk with your head held high and give praise to the Lord, even while you are walking in the eye of your storm. When the rain pours down on you, look, and see God's light through the dark clouds. God is the Alpha, the Omega *(Revelation 1:8, 1:11)*, the First and the Last *(Isaiah 44:6)*, the Author and Finisher of your faith. He is Abba Father, the Father to the fatherless. God is ALL around us!

I praise God for this story but most of all I thank Him for allowing me to share it with my loving friend, Jackie. I dedicate this story to her. God used Jackie on this particular stormy day, so my ears would hear what He was saying out of my own mouth. Learn to speak the word of God out of your mouth so you can hear His voice inside you. It was a wonderful experience and even more precious to me now because I was able to hear it from my own mouth, and not just in my head, writing it on a tablet of paper or typing it on the keyboard of my computer. Seeing the light through the darkness is not hard if your eyes are focused on the right person, God, and not yourself.

Please let us pray:

Father, I praise you for your goodness and your mercy. I praise you that you open our spirits to see who you are in the darkness. Lord, help us to see the victory and run the race. Father, we do not want to give Satan a chance to stop us from finishing the race. We run the race knowing we will finish because Jesus already won the battle. Thank you, Jesus, for you loved us before we were even born. Give us strength to focus and strength to run to the finish line. We get weary sometimes, Lord, when the storm pours on us and we cannot see the victory because of the clouds in our eyes. Father, remove the clouds so we can see clearly the victory. You, Lord, are our victory. You, Lord, are our prize. It is the prize of receiving you and the confidence in ourselves to run to your arms of mercy and grace. That is what we want to have, confidence to make it. I pray you will keep us moving forward and not backwards. To you, Lord, we give honor and glorify your name above all names. Thank you, Lord. Bless us and forgive us for being self-centered. Turn our heart and eyes back to you, oh God. Father, it is through your Holy Spirit we see clearly the right path to follow. We want to be in your will, Lord, walking to the finish line of glory. Thank you, Jesus. It is in Jesus' name we pray. Amen.

Randy B. Brown

Written By: Thelma Conway
19 March 1983

To My Beloved Daughter

As we look back through the years –
Some through smiles, some through tears
We know God hears our every prayer
And that His Son, Jesus, is always there!

Randy, you have been such a special joy to me
You have kept me straight when I wanted to flee!
Now, once again together, we go down the pathway of pain
But there IS sunshine on the other side of that lane.

You have been through many trials in your life
But, you are a good Mother, and an excellent Wife
Look back at all the good times you have had
Remember them always, honey, and forget the sad.

God is testing your strength, again today
Know He will be beside you, all along the way
He never puts on us more than He knows we can bear
In life, we have to take the load, and carry our share!

You will be well, you will be strong too
Because Jesus above, is looking out for you - -
I know it isn't easy – I have been there before
And sometimes I say: "Lord, I can't take anymore"

But, I know God hears my every cry and plea
I am wrapped in warmth that He loves you and me
Remember, when you are feeling not strong, alone and blue
Call on the Lord, and He will come to you!

It is hard to be a Mother, when our child is sick, we know
But I pray above for guidance and He shows me the way to go
I felt each time I went for Chemo – It was helping me to live
I found my strength in God and His Son, because I do believe

Each time left a Doctor's office, and I knew I was okay
I stopped and thanked the Lord first, before I went my way
Then I would go shopping, whether feeling good or bad
Because I got through another time, and I was surely glad!

It is a long road and it is up-hill all the way
But, honey, your Savior is there to help you today
So, ask God for strength to face each tomorrow
You will make it, because He will show you the pathway to follow

Keep your chin up – and keep your beautiful smile
For, truly, after all – life is so worthwhile!
Remember, your children and Allen will stand beside you - -
They will help you, my Daughter, to conquer this too!

Know everyone loves you – Daughter – and people still pray
That you will have the strength to get through each day!
Your Mom loves you so much – you are special, you see?
Call me when you need to talk honey, please come to me

With all my heart you're very special
and very dear to me. I love you so much! MOM

Grounded By the
Roots of Christ

(This story is dedicated to Stephen Powell)

It was a cool summer night on 12 September 2002. I was working in the back yard with my friend Steve, who had come over to help me get rid of bushes and trees I did not want around the house. Some trees were dead and some were still alive, but I did not like the looks of the landscape in my yard. While Steve was busy working on some vines that were hanging on the fence and I was raking them up, the Holy Spirit drew my eyes to a tall, dead, tree that was between us. I looked at Steve and said, "Steve! That tree right there is dead but it is still standing. How in the world can that tree stand when the whole thing is dead?" Steve said, "Because it is rooted in the ground!"

WOW! I thought that was amazing that the tree was totally dead, yet it was standing straight up as if it were alive. The roots we could not see were still good deep down in the ground so it was able to stand tall and straight as if it were still alive.

The Lord began to speak to me, and I started to tremble at the words I was hearing inside my spirit *(John 10:27)*. God showed me the tree had good roots deep in the ground, and because it was grounded so deep, it was able to stand. When we receive salvation, our souls become grounded, deeply rooted in Christ. God trims the dead branches of sin in our lives as we repent and then we can stand grounded by the roots of Christ deep within our spirits. Jesus is the vine and we are the branches. Apart from Him, we can do nothing *(John 15:5)*. God prunes us and reshapes our heart as we continue to grow in our walk and personal relationship with Him.

As Steve trimmed the branches before he pulled the tree out of the ground I watched in amazement at what the Lord had revealed to me. Our hearts are rooted in Christ. As we seek God's face *(Matthew 6:33)* by reading our Bible, going to church, fellowshipping with others, we will become rooted and grounded in the Lord Jesus Christ. We can start building our personal relationship with God and become vines with deep roots, standing tall like that tree. Because we ask in faith, believing what we talk to God in prayer about, He will hear our cries and will answer, for He is a loving and faithful God who never changes. God is the same today as He was yesterday *(Hebrews 13:8)*. Our souls will have deep roots that will hold us in the arms of Christ as we walk through the trials of life.

The Bible says that if you train up a child in the Lord, no matter what happens he will come back to the way of the Lord, because of the roots planted in his soul *(Proverbs 22:6)*. God becomes our deep roots, Jesus is the tree, and we are the branches on His tree of life. We may look dead to some because they know our past, but God sees deep within our heart. He is constantly trimming away the dead branches of sin in our lives by the convictions of the Holy Spirit *(John 3:17-18, Romans 8:1 and 1 Corinthians 11:32)*, not the condemnation of the enemy the world sees. We are rooted and grounded in Christ Jesus as we seek a closer personal relationship through prayer, and we get to know Him face to face.

Christ is the tree of life and we are the branches on the tree. We are grounded, rooted and stand, like the tree did, as we get to know Christ. Praying and talking with God just as if He were sitting next to you will build an intimate relationship with Him. We know, He will never leave us nor forsake us *(1 King 8:57 and Hebrews 13:5)*. Our hearts grow when the dead branches are cut off. The tree in my yard may be pulled up but because I am grounded in Christ my roots are deep and no one can take me from God's hand *(Romans 8:39 and John 10:29)*.

Trust and believe in the roots growing deep inside your soul and remember whom you belong to. Christ is our anchor and we want to be built on solid ground rooted in Him. God is the only true God. There are no others before him *(Jeremiah 10:10)*.

I want to be "Grounded By the Roots of Christ"! We are not dead in Christ but alive, rooted and grounded by the grace and mercy of God, our creator.

The tree is pulled out of the ground but the roots go on and on. We have to put stump killer on the roots to keep them from growing any more. Satan is a stump killer. He tries to kill our roots with the past sin in our lives. When we start encouraging ourselves in the Lord with the word of truth, we will grow stronger. We can do all things through Christ *(Philippians 4:13)*.

I thanked Steve for coming over and helping me on this night, because God uses people and things to give us revelations of Him. Tonight the Lord used Steve in my life to reveal His roots in my soul. I challenge you to look at people and things. Watch and see what is going on around you and let God reveal Himself to your spirit, personally. I love it when He reveals Himself to me. He is waiting for us to sit and talk with Him.

Pray, believing God will answer, because you are His child, saved by the Blood of Christ. Get grounded and rooted in the things of God, not the world. Look at things through the eyes of God and let Him reveal the unknown to you. The Lord has so much He wants to talk to us about, but we must be open to receive His voice any way

Randy B. Brown

He chooses to get our attention. His creation is the world. God will talk to us through His creation with revelations of Himself. Praise God for His mercy and grace. Praise Him for His unfailing love.

Let us pray:

My Heavenly Father, I know I am a sinner saved by the Blood of Jesus. I thank you for the grace and mercy you give to me. I thank you that I can be grounded and rooted in the Lord. As I pray, I will believe and trust that you will hear and answer because of my faith. Lord, build my faith. Increase the measure you give to me. Expand my measure so that my faith will be fully grounded and rooted in your love. Father, teach me to pray and talk with you as my personal, best friend. Father, I believe your word. I believe your ears hear my cries. I repent and ask you to trim the branches of sin off my life so I will have deeper roots in Christ. Thank you, Lord, for hearing my prayer. Thank you, Lord that you never leave me nor forsake me. Thank you, Lord that you are faithful and just. Father, I pray, asking in the mighty name of Jesus, the only true living Son of God. Thank you, Lord, for your grounding. Thank you for making my roots stronger in you, Lord. It is in the name of Jesus I pray and say thank you.

Written By: Thelma Conway
17 March 1993

Our First Great Grand-Child

On Friday, at 3:45 P.M., 5 March 1993 –
Another limb was added to our Family Tree.
A precious Great-Grandson arrived in our town,
Patiently we waited for you, Chase Andrew Brown!

Weighing 8 pounds, 7 ounces, for all the world to see
A sweetheart of a baby, we know you will be
You have stolen our heart, dear little boy
Oh how "Special" you are – and what a joy!

We love you so much, dear Great-Grandson –
Everyone's heart you have already won –
Please God, protect Chase from Heaven above
With your Blessed Caring and Special Love!

(Four GYN doctors and their nurses
got my granddaughter, Angel, through a difficult pregnancy
She was supposed to abort this child.
BUT GOD SAID NO! HE BELONGS TO ME
and
Chase Andrew Brown was delivered.
He is Gods Miracle!
and
Our Miracle Baby!

Simple Numbers on a Door

(This story is dedicated to JESUS)
(This is my Divine Healing Testimony)

On 27 February 2003, I sat in the hallway of the hospital, apprehensive about the impending results of my CAT scan. The Oncologist Surgeon was reviewing my results, determining the next step to take.

Three months earlier, on 23 November 2002, I was diagnosed with stage-four ovarian cancer. Exploratory surgery found cancer had spread throughout my body and the main tumor was inoperable. Nothing could be done. My family was called together and told there was no hope. Six weeks to six months left was all they could expect. A second opinion was no different. Chemotherapy was started as a last resort and Hospice was contacted. I was sent home with only a few weeks to live. Cancer. I knew what that was; I have had cancer before.

Cancer patients go through so much, having one surgery after another, test after test after test. Needles, blood work and chemo, but the cancer persists. Enduring all that pain and the outlook remains the same. I started chemo in December and now it was February. I hated the needles and the prospect of more surgery. Sitting in the hallway, pondering my options, wondering, did I want my few remaining weeks to be full of surgical pain, chemo side effects, and the prospects of endless needles?

If God takes me home soon, I have victory. If He leaves me here, I have victory. Tired and exhausted, I prayed for His will to be done, and strength to finish the race set before me. I was praying for His will to be done; at the same time, I was tired and needed His strength to finish this race set before me. I was scared, nervous and anxious, so many things were running through my mind as I sat there waiting to see the doctor.

To distract myself, I looked around, up and down the hallway. I noticed the room numbers. The door in front of me had the room number *"15171"*. Such a large number I thought. "Randy, let's talk about those numbers on the door," the Lord said. I felt a rush of comfort as he spoke my name.

As I sat there, He told me that the three *1's* represented the Father, the Son and the Holy Spirit and the 5 and 7 stood for me. Ever since I was a little girl, the numbers 5, 7, and 13 have been my 'favorite' numbers. The Lord knew the spiritual meaning of numbers fascinated me. However, where is my other favorite number 13? Wait, now I see it. I am 5 and 7; God is 1 in the center. 5+1+7= 13. There, right in the center of my life is God. I am again surrounded by the Holy Spirit and Jesus (1-5-1-7-1). Totally encased in the love of God. Right in front of me, all my favorite numbers, on one examining room door!

As I looked at the numbers, the Holy Spirit began to talk to me about my fear. He used those numbers to comfort my spirit. God explained that if I looked at how these numbers were placed, I would see my life is totally surrounded by His love, mercy, and grace. He has always been there, in all three persons, the Father, the Son, and the Holy Spirit. Taking care of me through out my life and not just this one trial. I was so comforted that my stomach stopped jumping, and I immediately calmed down. It felt as if God Himself was sitting right next to me, whispering in my ear. The Holy Spirit brought the presence of Jesus so close at that moment; I did not want to move, just sit there in his presence. Words cannot express the comfort of the Holy Spirit during times like this.

Finally, it was my turn to see the doctor. In the presence of the Lord, I walked in to receive my results. The CAT scan and the physical examination showed "marked improvement". Praise the Lord was the first thing out of my mouth. God did not leave me. He did not forsake me. His word is truth and He is faithful to His children.

Suddenly I realized the significance of the golden colored dust I had been seeing on me. For the past 8 months, gold dust had been appearing on my hands, on my face, and my neck. The Lord had been manifesting his presence to me in the form of gold dust. Here, in the hospital, it was all making sense. He surrounded me with my numbers, and physically showed his presence through the gold dust. God was doing something in me, but I did not know what until this moment. I knew God was about to do something even bigger in my life.

Romans 8:28 tells us that all things work together for those who are the called, and in God's time. God's time is not our time. We have to be patient and wait for His timing in the battles we are walking through. I praise God for giving me the revelation of those simple numbers on an examining room door. The gold dust was tangible proof of his love. It gave me comfort and freedom in my spirit. I was ready for whatever He wanted me to do to glorify the name of Jesus.

My surgery was scheduled for March 21, 2003. I was excited. It was also the first day of spring. The flowers begin to bloom, caterpillars come out of their cocoons as a butterfly, and people are fixing their yards for the summer. It is a new season, a fresh new beginning. I went into surgery with a positive attitude, but nothing could have prepared me for the surgeon's news when I woke up.

In the day-to-day world, we don't realize the depth of love from our friends and co-workers. It's during times like this when everyone pulls together to support you. God has put them there so he can speak through them, encouraging us. I have learned to receive God's love through that encouragement. It is all about faith, love, and unconditional love from others that God uses to help us get through those battles we fight. God does not give up on us; we cannot give up on ourselves. We must press through and make it to the finish line of glory.

My exploratory surgery in November showed cancer had spread to the liver, diaphragm, up into the abdomen, and down through the ovaries and tubes. A tumor the size of an orange, hung down in the midst of it all. The doctor went no further; the cancer was too wide spread for surgery to resolve anything. February's CAT scan showed the chemotherapy had shrunk the major tumor some, but the cancerous cells still remained where they were. It was now 3 weeks later. I had already lost too much weight, was too weak, and could not eat. I was wasting way from the chemotherapy. Surgeons wanted to remove as much cancer as they could, hoping to give me a few more months of quality life.

My youngest daughter, my son, and one of my best friends were in the surgical waiting room. Surgery was expected to last 5 long hours. Their hearts sank as the Surgeon came out one hour later. She's gone, they thought, she died on the table. The doctor approached, shaking his head. "Unbelievable," he said. "I have never seen anything like this in all my years of surgery. I looked, moved, poked, and prodded; there is no trace of cancer anywhere. I had to take the tubes and ovaries for the pathologist, but they looked absolutely normal." He looked at my family and friends, "I just can't believe it," he said in awe. "The tumor was gone, the cancer cells gone, everything looked normal. Everything was there three weeks ago, but now there is nothing. Not a trace of cancer anywhere."

God gave me a miracle.

For my follow up appointment, I went looking for the comfort of God around me. The numbers on the door again spoke to me. *"15151"*. All the numbers add up to *13,* my favorite number *5* in the middle of the *1's*, God, Jesus, and the Holy Spirit. From the left side, 1-5-1 = 7 the Holy Spirit, Me and God. From the middle to the right is 1-5-1 = 7 God, me and Jesus. There, once again, totally encased by God's love, comforting me with His unique ways of getting my attention. I knew everything was going to be okay again. Whatever the Lord wanted me to do I was ready to do it. I had no apprehension at all this time. I knew the results of the surgery; I was now waiting for the results of the pathology reports. Would they show hidden cancer cells?

I was concerned about having to continue with the chemotherapy treatments. God healed me, why should I go through more chemotherapy. The numbers on the door had comforted my spirit and I was ready for the doctor's decision. Knowing that God would guide the doctor's decisions, I would do what God wanted to glorify the name of His Only Son. The doctor told me even though I was healed, he still wanted me to complete the cycle of treatments. I was ready to do God's will. I knew He would be with me the whole time.

On the wonderful day when I took my last chemo treatment, my nurse and some of the office staff went outside with me to my car.

In the parking lot, we danced before the Lord with all of our heart, shouting praises to His name.

We walk through the battles pressing toward the goal *(Philippians 3:14)* for Jesus is our reward. Sometimes the battle is tough but as long as your heart is open to hear the voice of God inside you, anything is possible and the outcome is His victory! I knew God was in the middle of my life because of those simple numbers on a door. Whatever He wants to do through me, I want to be available to Him for His purposes. After all, He created me!

At the time of this writing, I am on the way to a full recovery with a great testimony of God's power through faith, prayer, love, and supernatural healing. Glory to Jesus, who made it all possible! Praise God for those simple numbers on an examining room door. He put them there to get my attention, so I would hear His voice speaking inside of me. God spoke I listened.

I encourage you to be open to the voice of the Lord and let God be the Lord of your life. He will speak to you in ways that will amaze you. Open up your heart to Him today and let Him show you great and mighty things that are hidden. That is what God wants to do with every one of us if we will just ask Him *(Jeremiah 33:3)*. If you do not know Jesus as your Lord and Savior, seek God, find a good Bible-teaching Holy-Spirit-filled church, so you will come to know Jesus. Get saved, by the blood He shed on the Cross for your sins that day at Calvary. It does not cost you anything, because God's grace of salvation is free to everyone. All you have to do is ask Him to come into your life and be your Savior, and then receive what you asked for in faith. God wants to reveal Himself to you in many unique ways, ways that are personal and intimate just between Him and you. He is no respecter of persons and He wants you to know Him intimately.

Open up your heart and receive Jesus today and live eternity in heaven.

I will not forget the closeness I felt that day. I knew the Lord was walking with me, through a very difficult time in my life. He is always there, waiting for us to call on Him. We must have an open heart so our ears can hear His voice. Through faith, we must believe that it will be done, in Jesus' name. Thank you, Father, for those simple numbers on a door that gave me so much comfort and peace from your heart to my heart!

Let us pray:

Father, thank you, for speaking to me in whatever way you know will get my attention. Lord, I pray that I will be open to hear your voice inside me in whatever way you choose to talk to me. You can use simple numbers on a door to speak to me for you know what will get my attention. Father, I thank you that you want to show me great and mighty things. Lord, these are things that show me who you are and things that will build my personal intimate relationship with you. Father, I thank you for Jesus who died on the Cross for my sins and gave me eternal life. Thank you for the Holy Spirit who gives me comfort and peace in this world. Lord, I ask that you make my anxious thoughts calm with your very voice inside me. I thank you, Lord, for the healings that come from your hand. Father, if I have to go through things to serve you, give me the strength to finish the battle that has already been won for me through your Son, Jesus. Keep me close to your side so I can feel your presence around me at all times. I will know I have nothing to fear because you have already taken care of it before I even began the trial. Thank you, Father, for victory in Jesus. Thank you, Lord, for your unconditional love. To Jesus I give all the honor and glory for the battle has been won and the victory is His. I pray in Jesus' name.

To end this book entitled <u>God Spoke I Listened</u>, I want to take the opportunity to invite you to meet my Jesus. If you do not know Jesus as you personal Savior, why don't you invite Him into your heart today? Receive Him as your Lord and Savior. Then build your personal, intimate relationship with the King of Kings! God wants to talk to you about so much if you will stop and listen to His voice inside you as you meet with Him every day.

Just say, "Jesus, I am a sinner and I ask you to forgive me of my sins. Come into my heart and be the Lord of my life. I receive you as my personal Savior and I believe, in faith, you are the only Son of God, who died on the Cross for all my sins. I believe, you were buried, and rose again. I receive your grace, mercy, and I thank you Jesus, for the gift of eternal life. In Jesus' name I pray."

Written By: Thelma Conway
17 May 1972

Lift Up Your Heart and Pray

There will be a little sunshine in your life every day
If you will just lift up your heart to God and pray –
For God loves us all and we glow with His love
As we ask for His help and healing powers from above.

Let me talk to you for a moment or two –
I will let you in on a secret, you and I know to be true
If we stop once a day, while at work or at play
To lift up our heart in joyous wonder to God and pray
He will help us like no one else could ever do
And He, alone, we know, will always pull us through!

So, when you feel tired, discouraged and full of torment
Look up to God, for His love will keep you content
We know our families stand beside us any way they can –
But, our God has loved us all since time began!

So let us put all our trust and faith in the Lord on high
And you will find that your troubles will never multiply
But, your troubles will go away and leave you feeling gay
For then you will know God has helped you in every way.

So, once again, I say "LIFT UP YOUR HEART AND PRAY"
And know God has taken all your troubles far away
There are greater days to come, bright days through the blue
For God is watching from above, and will always see you through.

ABOUT THE AUTHOR

Twice a victor over cancer, Randy Brown has a tremendous testimony of the goodness of God and His personal involvement in the lives of His children. Randy has experienced His dramatic intervention in her life, not only through divine healing, but also through her deep personal intimate relationship with Jesus. In the midst of many life challenges including "terminal" cancer, the Lord has visited Randy and shared His heart with her in dramatic visions and modern-day parables, which she shares with her readers in <u>God Spoke I Listened</u>. The Spirit of God has tabernacled with Randy, doing a dramatic work in her life, healing not only her physical body, but also the scars from years of abuse and rejection. Her book is a glorious testimony to the power of a mighty God!

The mother of three adult children and grandmother of ten, Randy has served the Lord for many years. She is on the Praise and Worship Team at River of Life Church in Jacksonville, North Carolina. She is a long-time member of the Daughters of Zion, a prophetic intercessory team covenanted to pray for Israel and the Jewish people. She has been an administrative assistant for the last 13 years of her 31 year career. Her powerful example of Christian character and fervor for the Lord has resulted in many being led to Christ and seeing their lives dramatically changed.

www.ingramcontent.com/pod-product-compliance
Lightning Source LLC
Chambersburg PA
CBHW020427290526
45785CB00002B/733